D0193939

CHILD
HEALTH

Dr. Miriam Stoppard

CHILD HEALTH

HEALTHCARE

DORLING KINDERSLEY

LONDON, NEW YORK, MUNICH,
MELBOURNE AND DELHI

DESIGN AND EDITORIAL   Kelly Flynn Associates

SENIOR MANAGING
ART EDITOR   Lynne Brown

MANAGING EDITOR   Jemima Dunne

SENIOR ART EDITOR   Karen Ward
SENIOR EDITOR   Penny Warren

PRODUCTION   Antony Heller

First published in Great Britain in 1998 by
Dorling Kindersley Limited, 80 Strand,
London WC2R 0RL
A Penguin Company

Reprinted 2001

Material in this publication was previously published
by Dorling Kindersley in *Baby and Child Health
Care* by Dr. Miriam Stoppard.

A CIP catalogue record for this book is available
from the British Library.
ISBN 0-7513-3611-4

Reproduced by Colourscan, Singapore and
IGS, Radstock, Avon
Printed and bound in the Slovak Republic
by Tlaciarne BB s.r.o., Banska Bystrica

See our complete catalogue at www.dk.com

Note: *We use the masculine pronoun "he" when
referring to the baby or child. This is for convenience and
clarity and does not reflect a preference for either sex.*

CONTENTS

INTRODUCTION 6
HOW TO USE THIS BOOK 8
A-Z OF COMPLAINTS 10

CHAPTER 1

CARING FOR A SICK CHILD 11

CALLING THE DOCTOR • TEMPERATURE
• MEDICINES • NURSING A SICK CHILD
• YOUR CHILD IN HOSPITAL

CHAPTER 2

INFECTIOUS DISEASES 23

DIAGNOSIS GUIDE 24

FEVER • CHICKENPOX • MEASLES • MUMPS
• GLANDULAR FEVER • RUBELLA • AIDS

CHAPTER 3

SKIN, HAIR AND NAILS 33

DIAGNOSIS GUIDE 34

ITCHING • CUTS AND GRAZES • BITES • BRUISE
• SPLINTER • INSECT STINGS • BLISTER • BURN
• SUNBURN • HEAT RASH • CHAPPING • CHILBLAINS
• BOIL • COLD SORE • NAPPY RASH • CRADLE CAP
• ECZEMA • HIVES • ATHLETE'S FOOT
• IMPETIGO • RINGWORM • LICE (NITS) • SCABIES
• INGROWING TOENAIL • VERRUCA

CHAPTER 4

EYES, EARS, NOSE, THROAT AND MOUTH 61

DIAGNOSIS GUIDE 62

COMMON COLD • CATARRH • SINUSITIS • SORE THROAT • TONSILLITIS • LARYNGITIS • GLUE EAR • EARACHE • OTITIS EXTERNA • EAR: FOREIGN BODY • NOSE: FOREIGN BODY • NOSEBLEED • STYE • STICKY EYE • CONJUNCTIVITIS • EYE: FOREIGN BODY • TEETHING • TOOTHACHE • MOUTH ULCER • GUM BOIL

CHAPTER 5

RESPIRATORY SYSTEM 83

DIAGNOSIS GUIDE 84

COUGH • BRONCHITIS • INFLUENZA • CROUP • HAYFEVER • ASTHMA • CHOKING • WHOOPING COUGH • COT DEATH

CHAPTER 6

DIGESTIVE SYSTEM 95

DIAGNOSIS GUIDE 96

COLIC • GASTROENTERITIS • FOOD POISONING • VOMITING • DIARRHOEA • CONSTIPATION • ENCOPRESIS • HERNIA • APPENDICITIS

CHAPTER 7

MUSCLES, BONES AND JOINTS 107

DIAGNOSIS GUIDE 108

SPRAIN • BROKEN BONE • LIMPING • GROWING PAIN

CHAPTER 8

NERVOUS SYSTEM 113

DIAGNOSIS GUIDE 114

DIZZINESS • HEADACHE • MIGRAINE • MENINGITIS

CHAPTER 9

URINARY AND REPRODUCTIVE SYSTEMS 119

DIAGNOSIS GUIDE 120

THRUSH • BALANITIS

USEFUL ADDRESSES 123
• GLOSSARY 124 • INDEX 126
• ACKNOWLEDGMENTS 128

INTRODUCTION

IT SEEMS ODD THAT THERE are so few books for parents that are devoted entirely to children's illnesses. Many baby books have a section on common childhood complaints, some even going so far as to include specific illnesses and their treatments; others approach the subject in a dictionary form, relying heavily on definitions but without giving very much background information and practical help to parents; very few indeed treat the subject with the kind of detail, explanations and guidelines that we have come to expect from similar books on adult diseases. Yet all parents worry about their children's health, and need the reassurance of a practical, easy-to-use guide: hence this book.

Over 80 common childhood complaints are arranged in separate chapters, by body system – for example, you will find bronchitis in the Respiratory System chapter while nosebleed and stye are in the Eyes, Ears, Nose, Throat and Mouth chapter – and form the mainstay of this book. All the information is given in simple terms which are easy to understand. Parents are directed to possible courses of action in a clear, logical way, with step-by-step advice. Emphasis on speed is always made when it is important to contact a doctor or call an ambulance. An at-a-glance A–Z index of complaints is also included for emergency use.

Most childhood illnesses are minor and others are easily preventable; inoculations are effective against most infectious diseases. In a baby, however, seemingly minor illnesses can cause complications: a cold that develops into a throat infection, for instance, may cause breathing difficulties. You will be understandably anxious if your child is sickening for something, is ill, or has had an accident. Sometimes deciding whether to seek medical help can be equally stressful. Even if your child's symptoms appear commonplace, you may worry that they are indicative of something more serious. You should never feel that you are being too cautious – if you find yourself wondering whether it is worth consulting the doctor, then

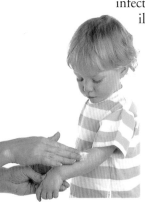

you probably should. However, to help you determine the most likely causes of a complaint, each entry contains an at-a-glance symptoms box giving the most common symptoms of that ailment. In addition, each chapter begins with a simple diagnosis guide, which also gives the most common symptoms of the complaints covered in the chapter.

Child Health has many useful illustrations; some will help with identification of symptoms, while others give practical tips in caring for a sick child. This is because one of my main aims is to give information in a readily accessible form, almost at a glance. There is, of course, ample opportunity to use the book as a straightforward reference book so that you gain knowledge gradually. But more than this, an anxious parent faced with a sick child in the middle of the night needs straightforward, uncomplicated information and advice, and I have, therefore, tried to arrange this book in a way that I would like to see if I found myself in that position as well.

· I don't have any personal axes to grind, but this book is opinionated and I make no apologies for this. However, where I have given an opinion, it is based on controlled research studies, or the lack of them, not on a purely personal basis.

Throughout the book, the main aim remains the same: to give you enough clear, up-to-date information, backed up by your own instincts, to know when to be your own family nurse or doctor and when it is essential to get specialist medical help.

How to Use This Book

When your child is ill, you need to know what to do – whether to call the doctor, or whether you can safely treat him at home yourself. You may also be unsure of what exactly is wrong with him and need help to determine the cause.

IF YOUR CHILD IS ILL AND YOU THINK YOU KNOW THE CAUSE

Turn to the relevant illness entry later in the book (use the special A-Z listing on page 10 for speed and ease of finding if you're in a hurry). There you will find an explanation of the ailment in question, together with a list of the symptoms most likely to appear. The circumstances under which you should call the doctor are clearly defined, and are followed by a section detailing the most probable treatment he will give. Most importantly, there is also advice on what you yourself can do to help your child.

If your child has an obvious symptom, but you are not sure which entry to look up, turn to the Diagnosis Guides at the beginning of each chapter. (All the complaints are listed according to the system affected – for example, bronchitis can be found in the Respiratory System chapter, while both nosebleed and stye are in the Eyes, Ears, Nose, Throat and Mouth chapter.) Although it can be difficult to make a diagnosis on the basis of only one or two symptoms, these guides should help to point you in the right direction.

IF YOU ARE LOOKING AFTER A SICK CHILD

The chapter Caring for a Sick Child on pages 11–22 gives tips on caring for your child when he is ill and shows, with illustrations, how to take a temperature and give medicines. It also provides practical

HOW TO USE THE ENTRIES

INTRODUCTION
Gives a description of the complaint, explaining why it arises and how it is likely to develop.

IS IT SERIOUS?
States whether or not the complaint is serious, and the conditions under which it would become serious.

WHAT SHOULD I DO FIRST?
Tells you how to determine whether he has a certain complaint or not; or it may suggest self-help measures that will provide relief while you contact the doctor. If the case is an emergency, the section will say so.

SEE ALSO
A cross-referencing system to other entries. You may be referred to another complaint because it could be the possible cause of the child's complaint.

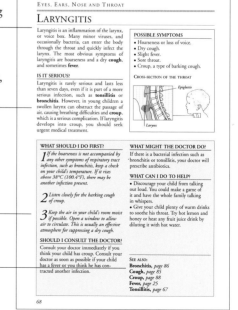

advice on how to reduce fevers and make your child comfortable, how and what to feed him, how to keep him amused and, should the need arise, how to prepare him for a stay in hospital.

USING THE ENTRIES

The illness entries are divided into a series of body-related chapters, and form the core of the book. They take two basic forms: in the majority of the entries, a detailed description of the illness is given, with a possible symptoms box for easy checking, a list of what to look for first and various treatments that might be given. In a few entries, where appropriate, no symptoms box is given since the symptom itself is the complaint's name – for instance, Dizziness in the Nervous System chapter. Two special entries (fever and vomiting) form the basis of so many common childhood illnesses,

that each one has a small symptoms chart of its own referring you on to the various possible causes.

Within each entry, another section, Should I Call the Doctor?, gives those instances where you should seek medical help and also defines the urgency of the assistance needed.

Emergency is just that, and you will be told to call an ambulance immediately or go straight to the nearest hospital casualty; *Consult your doctor immediately* also indicates urgency and you should get in touch with him, day or night to get his help; *Call your doctor as soon as possible* suggests some urgency but one that could await an early appointment during surgery hours; and lastly *Consult your doctor for advice* indicates that the ailment is not serious, but that it is advisable to talk to your doctor about it.

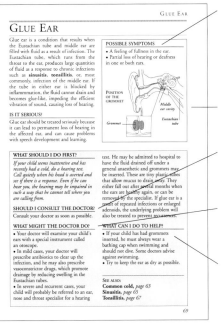

GLUE EAR

Glue ear is a condition that results when the Eustachian tube and middle ear are filled with fluid as a result of infection. The Eustachian tube, which runs from the throat to the ear, produces large quantities of fluid as a response to chronic infections such as **sinusitis**, **tonsillitis**, or, most commonly, infection of the middle ear. If the tube in either ear is blocked by inflammation, the fluid cannot drain and becomes glue-like, impeding the efficient vibration of sound, causing loss of hearing.

POSSIBLE SYMPTOMS
• A feeling of fullness in the ear.
• Partial loss of hearing or deafness in one or both ears.

POSITION OF THE GROMMET

Middle ear cavity

Grommet

Eustachian tube

IS IT SERIOUS?
Glue ear should be treated seriously because it can lead to permanent loss of hearing in the affected ear, and can cause problems with speech development and learning.

WHAT SHOULD I DO FIRST?
If your child seems inattentive and has recently had a cold, do a hearing test. Call quietly when his head is averted and see if there is a response. Even if he can hear you, the hearing may be impaired in such a way that he cannot tell where you are calling from.

SHOULD I CONSULT THE DOCTOR?
Consult your doctor as soon as possible.

WHAT MIGHT THE DOCTOR DO?
• Your doctor will examine your child's ears with a special instrument called an otoscope.
• In mild cases, your doctor will prescribe antibiotics to clear up the infection, and he may also prescribe vasoconstrictor drugs, which promote drainage by reducing swelling in the Eustachian tubes.
• In severe and recurrent cases, your child will probably be referred to an ear, nose and throat specialist for a hearing

test. He may be admitted to hospital to have the fluid drained off under a general anaesthetic and grommets may be inserted. These are tiny plastic tubes that allow mucus to drain away. They either fall out after several months when the ears are healthy again, or can be removed by the specialist. If glue ear is a result of repeated infections or enlarged adenoids, the underlying problem will also be treated to prevent recurrences.

WHAT CAN I DO TO HELP?
• If your child has had grommets inserted, he must always wear a bathing cap when swimming and should not dive. Some doctors advise against swimming.
• Try to keep the ear as dry as possible.

SEE ALSO:
Common cold, page 63
Sinusitis, page 65
Tonsillitis, page 67

69

POSSIBLE SYMPTOMS
Lists the symptoms that are likely to occur with the given complaint. Your child may have some or all of them; he may or may not develop them in the order given, although that is the most likely sequence.

DIAGRAMS
Show what to look for.

SHOULD I CONSULT THE DOCTOR?
Explains the circumstances under which you should seek medical assistance.

WHAT MIGHT THE DOCTOR DO?
Outlines the treatment most likely to be given to your child.

WHAT CAN I DO TO HELP?
Makes suggestions as to what a parent can do to assist the doctor in the treatment of the child, and gives home treatment and nursing tips.

A-Z GUIDE TO COMPLAINTS

Although the complaints covered in this book are listed according to the part of the body affected, there are times when it becomes important to be able to find something instantly. The handy A-Z index to each of the entries below should therefore be useful in a crisis.

To get the most from the book, once you have identified the complaint, read the entry through carefully, then follow the What Should I Do First? section to find out how best to proceed. If, after reading the entry, you are still not sure whether you know what is wrong with your child, don't hesitate: CALL YOUR DOCTOR. Even if it turns out to be something minor (it usually does!), it really is better to be safe than sorry; your doctor will never mind being contacted if you are uncertain about symptoms. If he does prescribe something for your child, always carry out his instructions absolutely precisely for the best and safest results.

INDEX OF COMPLAINTS

AIDS	32	Ear, foreign body in	72	Meningitis	118
Appendicitis	106	Earache	70	Migraine	117
Asthma	90	Eczema	51	Mouth ulcer	81
Athlete's foot	54	Encopresis	104	Mumps	29
		Eye, foreign body in	78		
Balanitis	122			Nappy rash	49
Bites	37	Fever	25	Nose, foreign body in	73
Blister	41	Food poisoning	99	Nosebleed	74
Boil	47				
Broken bone	110	Gastroenteritis	98	Otitis externa	71
Bronchitis	86	Glandular fever	30		
Bruise	38	Glue ear	69	Ringworm	56
Burn	42	Growing pain	112	Rubella	31
		Gum boil	82		
Catarrh	64			Scabies	58
Chapping	45	Hayfever	89	Sinusitis	65
Chickenpox	27	Headache	116	Sore throat	66
Chilblains	46	Heat rash	44	Splinter	39
Choking	92	Hernia	105	Sprain	109
Cold sore	48	Hives	53	Sticky eye	76
Colic	97			Stye	75
Common cold	63	Impetigo	55	Sunburn	43
Conjunctivitis	77	Influenza	87		
Constipation	103	Ingrowing toenail	59	Teething	79
Cot death	94	Insect stings	40	Thrush	121
Cough	85	Itching	35	Tonsillitis	67
Cradle cap	50			Toothache	80
Croup	88	Laryngitis	68		
Cuts and grazes	36	Lice (nits)	57	Verruca	60
		Limping	111	Vomiting	100
Diarrhoea	102				
Dizziness	115	Measles	28	Whooping cough	93

CARING FOR A SICK CHILD

Caring for a sick child can be a nerve-racking and frightening experience for any parent, yet it is one that nearly every one of us has to go through at one time or another. The secret of coping is knowledge – and in particular a commonsense understanding of what to do and when to do it, and when to call in the professionals. In the pages that follow, detailed basic information is given to enable you to make these decisions wisely, from how to read a temperature accurately once you have taken it, to how best to administer medicines to a wriggling baby or small child.

CALLING THE DOCTOR

Most parents seem to know instinctively when their child is sickening for something: the child may not be as lively as he usually is; he may refuse his food; he may become clingy. However, the parent is not always able to diagnose exactly what is wrong, nor is he or she necessarily able to recognize whether the child's symptoms are serious or not, or even potentially serious. An ill child is always a distressing sight and the situation can be made even more tense if you cannot decide whether or not to call out the doctor.

There are some circumstances, for example after a serious injury, when medical help should be sought immediately. For most parents, these situations are quite obvious. There are, however, many more situations where the seriousness isn't as clear-cut. This is where the worry comes in: "Are my child's symptoms quite normal or are they potentially serious?" What you must remember is that most doctors will not mind if you seek their advice. Always follow your instincts and, if you are ever in doubt, contact your doctor.

If your child is already undergoing treatment from your doctor and you are worried about his progress, call your doctor again. Don't take your child to the nearest casualty department, because the medical staff in the casualty department will not be able to change any of your child's treatment without consulting your own doctor first.

Your sick child will need lots of reassuring cuddles.

WHEN TO CALL YOUR DOCTOR

Listed below are the circumstances under which you should always call your doctor. The following are all important signs so never ignore them.

Temperature
• A raised temperature of over 39°C (102.2°F).
• A raised temperature accompanied by drowsiness and a purplish rash, plus any other obvious signs of illness.
• A raised temperature accompanied by a convulsion or if your child has had convulsions in the past.
• A raised temperature accompanied by a stiff neck and headache.
• A temperature below 35°C (95°F) accompanied by a cold skin surface, drowsiness, quietness and listlessness.
• A temperature that drops and then rises again suddenly.
• A temperature of more than 38°C (100.4°F), for more than three days.

Diarrhoea
• If your baby has diarrhoea for more than six hours.
• If diarrhoea is accompanied by pain in the abdomen, a temperature or any other obvious signs of illness.

Vomiting
• If your baby has been vomiting for more than six hours.
• Prolonged, violent vomiting.
• Dizziness plus nausea and headaches.
• Nausea and vomiting accompanied by right-sided pain in the abdomen.

Loss of appetite
• If your baby goes off his food suddenly, or is less than six months old and doesn't seem to be thriving.
• If your child usually has a hearty appetite, but refuses all food for a day and seems listless.

Pain and discomfort
• If your child has headaches and feels sick and dizzy.
• If your child complains of blurred vision, especially if he's recently had a bang on the head.
• If your child has severe griping pains, which occur at regular intervals.
• If your child has a pain in the right side of his abdomen and feels sick.

Breathing
• If his breathing is laboured and his ribs draw in sharply with each breath.

EMERGENCIES

Always get your child to the nearest hospital by ambulance or car if you notice any of the following:
• Your child has stopped breathing.
• Your child is breathing with difficulty and his lips are going blue.
• Your child is unconscious.
• Your child has a deep wound that is bleeding badly.
• Your child has a serious burn (see p. 42).
• Your child has a suspected broken bone (see p. 110).
• Your child has a chemical in his eyes.
• Your child's ear or eye has been pierced.
• Your child has been bitten.
• Your child has eaten a poisonous substance.

TEMPERATURE

In children, normal body temperature ranges from 36°C (96.8F) to 37°C (98.6°F). Any temperature over 37.7°C (100°F) is classed as a fever. Hypothermia develops if the temperature falls below 35°C (95°F). Body temperature will vary according to how active your child has been and the time of day: it is lowest in the morning because there is little muscle activity during sleep, and highest in the late afternoon after a day's activity. An abnormally hot forehead could be the first indication you have that your child has a temperature. To be accurate, however, you must take your child's temperature with a thermometer. Because the temperature control centre in the brain is primitive in young children, the temperature can shoot up more rapidly than in adults. When a fever is present, you should take your child's temperature again after 20 minutes, just in case it was only a transitory leap. Never regard a high temperature as the only accurate reflection of whether your child is ill or not; a child can be very ill without a high temperature or quite healthy with one.

THERMOMETERS

There are three main types of thermometer: *mercury, digital* and *liquid crystal.*

Mercury thermometers are the most accurate means of assessing a temperature. Made of glass, they register the temperature when the mercury expands up the tube to a point on the scale. There are two different ways to take a child's temperature with a mercury thermometer: for a younger child take it under his armpit; from about six or seven you can take it orally, as long as you can trust him not to bite the thermometer. To read a mercury thermometer, hold it between your finger and thumb and turn until you can see the point on the scale.

Digital thermometers are easy to use with children of all ages and are safer than mercury thermometers to use orally since

---

TIPS FOR TAKING TEMPERATURE

- Never take your child's temperature if he has just stopped running about.
- Never leave your child alone with a thermometer in his mouth.
- If there is an accident and a mercury thermometer breaks in your child's mouth, remove the pieces of glass quickly and carefully. The mercury is unlikely to spill from its tube but if it does, tell your child to spit out as much as he can; mop up the rest with a dry tissue. If he swallows any mercury, call your doctor.
- Make sure there is no break in the mercury inside the thermometer – it will affect the reading.
- If your thermometer is cracked, throw it away immediately.

---

they are unbreakable. Digital thermometers are battery-operated, so be sure to keep spare batteries on hand.

Liquid crystal thermometers have a heat-sensitive panel on one side and panels with numbers on the other side. When the sensitive side is placed on the forehead, the numbers (your child's temperature) light up. Liquid crystal thermometers are not as accurate as mercury or digital thermometers but are safe and easy to use.

TREATING A RAISED TEMPERATURE

The raised temperature that accompanies an illness is the body's way of responding to infection, and is a sign that the body is marshalling its defences (see p. 25). If your child has a high temperature, he will be very uncomfortable and irritable, so it is important that you lower his temperature. To do this, remove your child's clothes and blankets, and leave him covered by only a single cotton sheet. If his temperature rises above 39°C (102°F), he could be more comfortable left uncovered but wearing a short-sleeved cotton T-shirt and underpants or a vest and nappy.

If your child's temperature is over 39°C (102.2°F) for longer than half an hour, and removing his bedclothes hasn't helped, try tepid sponging, starting from the top of his head and working your way down his whole body (see p. 26).

The most efficient way of reducing your child's fever is to give him medicine. Paracetamol is probably the best choice with children, as it has few side effects. It also has the advantage of being easily available in liquid form, so it is much easier to give to young children. Do not give it to your child for longer than two days without consulting your doctor.

USING MERCURY AND DIGITAL THERMOMETERS

Always wash a thermometer with cool water after it has been used. Never wash a mercury thermometer in hot water because this can cause the glass to crack. Always store a thermometer in its own case and in an accessible place after use.

ARMPIT METHOD
Use a mercury thermometer for this method if possible.

1 Hold the thermometer by the top end and shake it down sharply until the mercury falls below the 35°C (95°F) mark. Sit with your child on your lap, facing away from you. With the thermometer in your right hand, raise your child's left arm so that you expose the armpit.

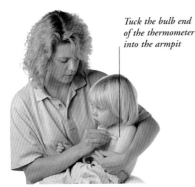

Tuck the bulb end of the thermometer into the armpit

2 Put the thermometer into the armpit and lower his arm over it. Hold the arm down for two minutes (or according to manufacturer's instructions), remove and read.
Note *The reading when taken in the armpit will be about 0.6°C (1°F) lower than the child's actual body temperature.*

USING AN ORAL THERMOMETER
Use a digital thermometer for this method if possible.

1 Ask your child to open his mouth and raise his tongue. Place the thermometer under it.

2 Ask your child to place the tip of his tongue firmly behind his lower front teeth – this will hold the thermometer in place. Then ask him to close his lips – but not his teeth – over it.

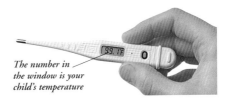

The number in the window is your child's temperature

3 Leave the thermometer in your child's mouth for two minutes (or according to the manufacturer's instructions), remove and read the number in the window.

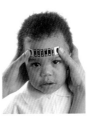

USING A LIQUID CRYSTAL STRIP THERMOMETER
Carefully position the heat-sensitive side on your child's forehead – the temperature should light up on the outside of the strip.

MEDICINES

When you take your child to the doctor he may prescribe some form of medicine for him. Ask your doctor to give you as much information as possible about the medicines: ask if there are likely to be any side effects, whether there are foods that should be avoided or special precautions that should be observed while your child is taking the medication, and clarify whether to give the medicine before or after a meal.

Most medicines for young children are made up in a sweetened syrup to make them more palatable, and can be given with a spoon, tube or dropper. Droppers and tubes are often more suitable for babies who

haven't learnt to swallow from a spoon. Some medicines for older children are supplied as tablets or capsules.

On most occasions your child will be co-operative but there may be the odd occasion when he simply refuses to take his medicine. It is very important that your child takes the medicine prescribed when he is ill. In fact, I think that this is one occasion when blackmail is justified. So don't hesitate to give the medicine with ice cream or another favourite food. Very occasionally a child will resist physically. When this happens, there really is no alternative but for you to be forceful.

GIVING MEDICINES TO A BABY OR YOUNG CHILD

It can be more difficult to administer medicines to babies because they wriggle. You will need the help of another adult or older brother or sister. Position your

baby carefully so that he is slightly raised. Never lay him down flat while giving him medicine because he may inhale the medicine into his lungs.

USING A SPOON

1 If the baby is very young, sterilize the spoon by boiling it or placing it in a sterilizing solution. Hold your baby in the crook of your arm. If he won't open his mouth, open it by gently pulling down his chin; if necessary get someone else to do this.

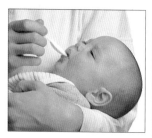

2 Place the spoon on his lower lip, raise the angle of the spoon and let the medicine run into his mouth.

USING A DROPPER

1 Hold your baby as described left and take up the specified amount of medicine into the glass tube.

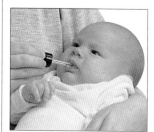

2 Place the dropper in the corner of your baby's mouth and release the medicine gently.

USING A MEDICINE TUBE

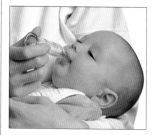

Pour the required dose into the tube. Hold your baby as described far left. Place the mouth-piece on his lower lip and let the medicine trickle into his mouth.

OTHER METHODS
Measure the required dose into a container, dip your little finger into it, then let your baby suck it off your finger. A plastic syringe can also be helpful. Ask your doctor or pharmacist to give you one.

GIVING MEDICINES AND TABLETS TO OLDER CHILDREN

On the whole, children do not generally mind medicine too much and often want to pour medicine out for themselves rather than let you give it to them. I have listed a few tips, below, that may help if your child is difficult. For example, tablets can be crushed and mixed with jam or ice-cream. Capsules, however, should not be broken.

It is very important that your child takes his medicine exactly as prescribed

TIPS FOR GIVING MEDICINES

Giving medicines to babies
• Enlist the help of another adult or older brother or sister.
• If you are on your own, wrap a blanket around your baby's arms so that you can stop him struggling and hold him steady.
• Only put a little of the medicine in his mouth at a time.
• If your baby spits the medicine out, get the other person to hold his mouth open while you carefully trickle the medicine into the back of his mouth. Then, gently but firmly, close his mouth.

Giving medicines to older children
• Suggest that your child holds his nose while taking the medicine, so lessening the effect of the taste.
• Don't forcibly hold your child's nose, as he may inhale some of the medicine.
• Mix liquid medicine with another syrup such as honey.
• Don't add liquid medicine to a drink, as it will just sink to the bottom of the glass or stick to the sides and you won't be sure that your child has had the whole dose.
• Show your child that you have his favourite drink ready to wash the taste of the medicine away; do this even if you do not normally allow him to have this drink.
• Help your child to clean his teeth after taking any liquid medicine to prevent syrup sticking to his teeth.
• Crush tablets between two spoons and mix the powder with something sweet, such as honey, jam or ice-cream.

MEDICINES

GIVING DROPS

Ear, nose or eye infections are generally treated with external drops. It is always easier to administer drops to a baby or young child if you lay him on a flat surface before you begin and enlist some help to keep him still and hold his head steady. An older child will probably be more co-operative and you will only need to ask him to tilt his head back or to the side, while you put the drops in.

EAR DROPS

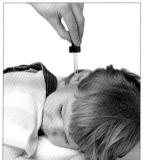

1 Carefully lay your child on his side with the affected ear uppermost. (If you have a young baby, hold him in your arms.) Gently and slowly let the drops fall into the centre of his ear.

2 Hold your child steady until the drops have run into the canal.

NOSE DROPS

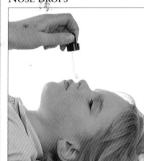

1 Tilt your child's head back and drop liquid into each nostril. (If you have a young baby, hold him in your arms.)

2 Count the number of drops as you put them in. Two or three at a time are normally sufficient; any more will run down his throat and could cause him to cough and splutter.

EYE DROPS

1 Tilt your child's head so that his affected eye is lowermost. (If you have a young baby, hold him in your arms.) If this is difficult, get someone to hold him while you administer the drops.

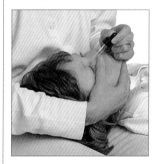

2 Very gently pull his lower eyelid down and let the drops fall between his eye and his lower lid.

TIPS FOR GIVING DROPS

• Warm nose drops and ear drops by standing the container in a bowl of warm, *not hot*, water for a few minutes, so that your child doesn't get too much of a shock when the liquid drops into his nose or ear.
• Be careful not to let the dropper touch your child's nose, ear or eye, or you will transfer the germs back to the bottle.

If the dropper *does* touch your child, make sure you wash it thoroughly before putting it back in the bottle.
• Proprietary drops should not be used for longer than three days without consulting a doctor – if they are used for too long, they can cause worse irritation and inflammation than the condition you were treating in the first place.

MEDICINE CHEST

You should always keep some medicines in the house in case of emergency in the middle of the night when you may not be able to get to a chemist easily. Keep them somewhere obvious so that you can find them quickly when you need them. Never mix different pills up in the same container and never keep any left-over prescription medicines. Keep all medicines well out of reach of children, in a high, locked cupboard, if necessary. You should also have a first-aid kit. Keep all the equipment in a clean, dry, airtight box and put it somewhere it can be found in an emergency.

The items listed below would all be useful to have in emergencies and are therefore well worth keeping in the house.

Medicines to avoid

The following items, commonly given as useful, should be avoided:

• Any proprietary product containing a local anaesthetic, such as amethocaine or lignocaine, because they can cause allergies. They are most generally found in creams for mouth ulcers or insect stings.
• Any skin creams containing antihistamines (unless prescribed by your doctor); they can cause skin allergies.
• Any proprietary product that contains aspirin.
• Mouth washes, gargles, eye drops, nose drops and ear drops, unless recommended by your doctor.

MEDICINE CABINET

• Mercury, digital or liquid crystal thermometer – keep two for safety.
• Junior paracetamol tablets.
• Liquid paracetamol – infants: from three months to six years or junior: from six to twelve years.
• Calamine lotion.

First-aid Kit
• Box of adhesive dressings.
• Wound dressings – cotton wool and gauze pad already attached to a bandage.

• Mild antiseptic wipes.
• Cotton wool.
• Mild antiseptic cream.
• Gauze dressings – keep dry and paraffin-coated ones.
• Surgical tape.
• Crepe bandages for supporting sprains and strains.
• Open-weave bandages.
• Triangular bandage.
• Safety pins, scissors and blunt-edged tweezers.

USEFUL HOUSEHOLD ITEMS

• Packet of frozen peas, or ice cubes in plastic bags for cold compresses.
• Newspaper, folded it can make a splint.
• Elastic belt to support a strain/sprain.
• Rehydration fluid to replace fluid lost after vomiting or diarrhoea.

• Bicarbonate of soda to add to a bath to relieve itching.
• Salt to add to a bath to clean wounds and deter infection.
• Vinegar to mix with water to soothe jellyfish stings.

NURSING A SICK CHILD

Few parents escape being called upon to look after a sick child – all children fall ill at some time. Babies often become very clingy and may cry more than normal because they do not understand what is happening to them. If a baby is being breastfed he will probably want to be fed more often, for the comfort of being near you as much as anything else. Bottle-fed babies will also want to be cuddled and will want smaller feeds more often. If your baby has recently given up his bottle, you may find that he wants it back again.

Older children can also become rather insecure when they are ill and often want to be with a parent all the time. Nursing a child does not require any special skills or techniques, just love and patience. Simply use your common sense. If you are worried, take your child to your doctor (see pp. 12–13) or ask for a home visit. If any medicines are prescribed, make sure you give them exactly as directed and follow any nursing tips your doctor gives you.

SHOULD MY CHILD STAY IN BED?

Take your lead from your child about whether to keep him in bed or not. There's no real need to keep a child with a fever in bed, although he should stay in a draught-free room where the temperature is kept constant. The room does not have to be particularly hot – if it is comfortable for you, it should be warm enough for him. If your child is really ill, he will probably want to stay still and will sleep a lot but when he is awake he will want to be with you – make up a bed for him in the room where you are working so that he can see and hear you. If he wants to be out of bed and playing, let him do so in the corner of the room. Leave his bed straightened so that he can go there when he wants to. If he is very tired, it is better to put him to bed, but remember to visit him regularly so that he does not feel neglected.

TIPS FOR NURSING YOUR CHILD
• Use cotton sheets – they are much more comfortable for a child with a temperature.
• Change his sheets regularly, particularly if he has a fever – clean sheets feel better.
• Let him get up if he does not want to stay in bed all the time but put a jumper on over his pyjamas, and make sure he's wearing socks or slippers.
• Leave a box of tissues on his bedside table.
• Leave a bowl beside your child's bed if he is feeling sick so that he doesn't have to run to the toilet. If he vomits, hold his head and comfort him, and give him a strongly flavoured sweet, or help him clean his teeth, to take away the after-taste.

SHOULD I ISOLATE MY CHILD?

Most evidence suggests that, in cases of infectious diseases, the degree of severity of the disease increases if there has been sustained close contact. It is, therefore, advisable to keep other children away from the infected child as much as possible. Obviously, if your child has a more serious infection that needs isolation, such as meningitis (see p. 118), your doctor will arrange for him to be admitted to hospital or advise you on the necessary precautions. If your child has rubella (see p. 31), you should warn any women you think may be pregnant – or who may come in contact with someone who is pregnant.

FEEDING A SICK CHILD

Most children with a fever don't want to eat, so while you should offer food, you should never force your child to eat if he seems unwilling. As long as he is getting plenty of liquid, he can survive perfectly well for two or three days on very little. When the illness is over, your child's appetite will return. As soon as it does, take advantage of it and let him eat as heartily as he wants to.

GETTING A SICK CHILD TO DRINK

While your child can survive without much food when he is ill, it is important that he drinks as much as possible to replace any fluid lost in sweating and vomiting or diarrhoea. A fevered child needs to drink at least 100–150ml (3–5fl oz) liquid per kilo (2lb) of body weight per day, or 200ml (7fl oz) per kilo (2lb) if he is vomiting or has diarrhoea. Get him to drink as often as you can; help an older child by leaving his favourite drink by the bed. Fizzy glucose drinks are neither nutritious nor necessary; I do not recommend them.

OCCUPYING A SICK CHILD

When your child is ill you can legitimately spoil him. Let him play with games that previously have never been allowed in bed. Even messy activities like painting will not cause too much mess if you put a large sheet of polythene over the bed.

Be easy on yourself as well and relax all the rules on tidiness – you can always clear up later. Sit down and spend time with him: read him stories, play games or help him with his colouring. Let him watch television while he is ill – have the television in his room or in the room where you are both sitting. Buy him some new toys. If he isn't too ill, wrap them and play a game with the parcel; ask him to guess what's in it and let him tear off the wrapping. Ask his friends to come and see him and let them play for a short time. If your child is not in bed all the time, there's absolutely no reason to keep him indoors on a warm day, even if he has a mild fever, but don't let him exercise too strenuously. If he wants to stay outside for longer than a few minutes, he is probably getting better anyway.

FEEDING AND DRINKING TIPS
Feeding your child
• Give your child small meals more often than you would normally.
• Don't scold him for not eating – he will eat again as soon as he gets better.
• Give your child his favourite foods.
• If your child has a sore throat, give him ice-cream or an ice lolly made with fruit juice or yoghurt to soothe it.
• If your child is feeling slightly sick, give him mashed potato.

Making drinks more interesting
• A sure ploy is to offer drinks in a tiny glass or egg cup. It is more fun and makes the quantities look smaller.
• Give your child fresh fruit juices and dilute them with fizzy mineral water to make them more fun.
• Use an interesting straw such as a curly or bendy one.
• If your child does not like milk, make it more attractive by adding milkshake mixes or ice-cream.
• Vary the drinks as much as possible.
• With a young child or baby, get him to sip drinks from a teaspoon. You could make it seem like a game by using a long-handled spoon.

GETTING BETTER

As your child gets better his appetite will start to come back and he will probably be more active. As soon as his temperature is back to normal in the morning and evening, he is probably ready to go back to school, although, if he has been suffering from an infectious illness, it may be wise to check with your doctor first. A young child may have regressed slightly while he was ill. For example, if he was just out of nappies you may have to start potty training again. Try not to worry about this too much.

YOUR CHILD IN HOSPITAL

You will be doing your child a great favour if you encourage him to think about hospitals as friendly places. Try to take him with you if you are visiting a family friend or relative – provided the person does not mind and visiting regulations allow it.

PREPARING YOUR CHILD

If your child has to go into hospital, for an operation, for example, and you are given some warning, prepare him by discussing as many aspects of his stay as possible. Talk about it with the rest of the family as well and get him generally used to the idea.

Answer all his questions honestly. Don't make promises that you can't keep and don't tell lies. If he is having an operation, he will probably ask you if there will be any pain or discomfort after the operation. If you say that nothing is going to hurt and it does, he will simply get a shock and will not trust you again in the future. Explain that there will be some discomfort but that it won't last long.

Another good way to prepare him for a hospital stay is to read him a book about someone who goes into hospital. You could also buy him a toy stethoscope and play doctors and nurses with him. Encourage him to be the doctor or nurse and suggest that he makes up a hospital bed for his favourite teddy bear or toy.

IN HOSPITAL

Few children's wards are frightening places. However, hospitals have found that it is very important for parents to be with their children as much as possible while they are in hospital and, because of this, almost all now allow parents to stay with their child, particularly if he is very young. Many hospitals have sleeping facilities for parents with children up to the age of six.

When you are there, ask the ward sister and nurses how you can help with the daily routine. You will be encouraged to bath and change your child, and to help with his feeding. You can read books and play games with him and any other children in the ward who want to join in. If the ward has a teacher, ask if you can help with your child's schoolwork. If he is well enough and will be in hospital for a while, ask his own teacher to give you the work he would normally be doing at school.

If you cannot be with your child all day, try to arrange a rota so that someone he knows well is with him all the time.

BACK HOME FROM HOSPITAL

It's quite normal for a child to behave a little oddly when he comes out of hospital. Firstly, your child's sleeping and eating patterns may have changed. Hospital meals, and certainly bedtimes, tend to be earlier than you'd have them at home. Secondly, because your child has been away from his domestic discipline, you may find that he will make a fuss about small points like brushing his teeth. Don't be too hard on him at first, give him time to readjust to being at home before you insist that he fits in with the old routine.

WHAT TO TAKE INTO HOSPITAL

If you can, you and your child should pack his case together a few days before he has to go in.

- Three pairs of pyjamas.
- Dressing gown and slippers.
- Three pairs of ankle socks.
- Hair brush and comb.
- Sponge bag with soap, flannel, toothbrush, toothpaste.
- Bedside clock.
- Portable radio or cassette player with headphones.
- Favourite books and portable games.
- Favourite picture or photograph to put by his bedside.

CHAPTER 2

INFECTIOUS DISEASES

Infectious childhood illnesses are less common
than they once were, thanks to the availability of
immunization, but they still occur and it is still
agonizing to have to cope with a bored, uncomfortable
child going through the discomforts of measles,
mumps, rubella or chickenpox – even when you
know that they are not life-threatening. In the
pages that follow, these and other common
infectious diseases are described in detail, with a
wealth of down-to-earth advice to enable you
to help your child through them.

DIAGNOSIS GUIDE

Children will always catch infectious diseases, so it is important to be able to identify and treat them when they occur. To use this section, look for the symptom most similar to the one that your child is suffering from then turn to the relevant entry. See also p. 13 for a useful list of emergency symptoms.

BLOTCHY RED RASH
starting behind the ears and spreading elsewhere, with swollen neck glands *possibly* **Rubella**, see p. 31

RED-BROWN RASH
starting behind the ears and spreading elsewhere, usually preceded by runny nose and sore eyes *possibly* **Measles**, see p. 28

ACHES AND PAINS
with swollen glands and a rash behind the ear *possibly* **Glandular fever**, see p. 27

INTENSELY ITCHY SMALL BLISTERS
in clusters on the trunk then the rest of the body *possibly* **Chickenpox**, see p. 27

HEADACHE
with fever and a rash *possibly* **Measles**, see p. 28 or **Chickenpox**, see p. 27

SWELLING ON EITHER OR BOTH SIDES OF THE FACE *possibly* **Mumps**, see p. 29

SWOLLEN NECK GLANDS
with sore throat accompanied by a fever possibly **Glandular fever**, see p. 30, or **Tonsillitis**, see p. 67

FEVER

A fever is a temperature of 37.7°C (100°F) or over. Consult your doctor if your baby's temperature remains high in spite of tepid sponging (see p. 26). Consult your doctor immediately if your child's temperature is as high as 39°C (102.2°F).

ACCOMPANYING SYMPTOMS	COMMON CAUSES
Your child has a cough and a runny nose.	He possibly has a **Common cold**, p. 63.
Your child has a cough, sore throat and aches and pains.	He possibly has **Influenza**, p. 87.
Your child has a sore throat and difficulty in swallowing.	He may have **Tonsillitis**, p. 67. If his voice is hoarse, he may have **Laryngitis**, p. 68. If his neck glands are swollen, he may have **Glandular fever**, p. 30.
Your child has a rash of itchy, red spots starting on the trunk.	He may have **Chickenpox**, p. 27.
Your child had a runny nose and sore eyes and now has a brownish-red rash.	He possibly has **Measles**, p. 28.
The sides of your child's face and the area under his chin are swollen.	He possibly has **Mumps**, p. 29.
Your child's ears are painful, or, if he is too young to tell you, he cries and tugs at his ear.	He possibly has a middle ear infection or **Earache**, p. 70.
Your child has diarrhoea.	He could have **Gastroenteritis**, p. 98 or **Food poisoning**, p. 99.
Your baby or child is breathing rapidly and with great difficulty.	CONSULT YOUR DOCTOR IMMEDIATELY Your child may have **Bronchitis**, p. 86 or **Croup**, p. 88.
Your child cannot bend his neck without pain, and turns away from bright light.	CONSULT YOUR DOCTOR IMMEDIATELY Your child may have **Meningitis**, p. 118.

Continued on next page

FEVER: CONTINUED

The range of normal body temperature is 36–37°C (96.8–98.6°F). Anything over 37.7°C (100°F) is a fever, although the height a temperature reaches is not necessarily an accurate reflection of the seriousness of the sickness. A fever is not in itself an illness, but rather is a symptom of one (see p. 25). Apart from any illness, your child's temperature will reflect the time of day and activity level: after a very strenuous game of football, for example, the temperature could temporarily be over 38°C (100.4°F).

IS IT SERIOUS?

A temperature of over 37.7°C (100°F) is always serious in a baby under six months old. If the temperature remains high, there is also a slight risk of a convulsion occurring.

WHAT SHOULD I DO FIRST?

1 If you suspect that your child has a fever, take his temperature (see p. 15), then check it again 20 minutes later.

2 Put your child to bed, remove most of his clothing and cover only with a light sheet, even if the room is cool.

3 Lower a temperature of over 40°C (104°F) by sponging your child all over with tepid water (it should be comfortable to the inside of your wrist). To do this, wring out a flannel or sponge in tepid water so that it is still dripping. Starting from the head, and using gentle strokes, sponge the whole of your child's body. Change the flannel or sponge when it feels warm.

4 Check the temperature every five minutes and stop tepid sponging when it drops to 38°C (100.4°F). Never sponge your child with cold water as this will cause his blood vessels to constrict, preventing heat loss and therefore increasing his temperature.

5 Give paracetamol only if other methods of reducing the fever have failed. Never give aspirin to a child under the age of 12, particularly if he has the symptoms of chickenpox or influenza.

6 Encourage your child to drink small amounts of fluid at regular intervals to prevent dehydration.

SHOULD I CONSULT THE DOCTOR?

Consult your doctor immediately if your child is under six months old. Consult him immediately if your child has a convulsion, has had a convulsion in the past, or if they run in the family; if the fever lasts for more than 24 hours; or if you are worried about any of the other symptoms.

WHAT MIGHT THE DOCTOR DO?

If the underlying cause is bacterial infection, antibiotics will probably be prescribed. If it is an ailment like chickenpox, or **common cold**, then no medication will be given, just advice on how to make your child comfortable.

WHAT CAN I DO TO HELP?

• Place a cold compress or a wet facecloth on your child's forehead.
• Don't wake your child to take his temperature. Sleep is more important.

SEE ALSO
Chickenpox, page 27
Common cold, page 63
Influenza, page 87
Measles, page 28

CHICKENPOX

Chickenpox is a very common, infectious childhood disease. It has an incubation period of between 17 and 21 days and causes only mild symptoms. Some sufferers may have a headache and a fever, though the majority give no real indication of illness at all except for the characteristic itchy chickenpox spots. The spots cover most parts of the body and can even appear in the mouth, anus, vagina or ears. They develop every day for three to four days and quickly create tiny **blisters** that leave a scab. Your child is infectious until the scabs have dropped off. The spots may leave shallow scars when they heal if the child scratches them too vigorously.

IS IT SERIOUS?

Chickenpox is not a serious illness. However, in rare cases, the chickenpox virus may cause encephalitis or be complicated by Reye's syndrome.

POSSIBLE SYMPTOMS

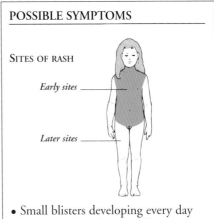

SITES OF RASH

Early sites

Later sites

- Small blisters developing every day for three to four days, usually starting on the trunk, then spreading to the face, arms and legs, and eventually scabbing over.
- Intense itchiness.
- Headache and fever.

WHAT SHOULD I DO FIRST?

1 Damp down the itchiness by applying calamine lotion to the rash, or by giving your child warm baths in which you have dissolved a handful of bicarbonate of soda.

2 As far as possible, keep your child away from other children; don't send him to school until the scabs have all dropped off.

SHOULD I CONSULT THE DOCTOR?

Consult your doctor as soon as possible to confirm that your child has chickenpox. Consult him if the spots develop redness with swelling, which indicates infection, or if your child is unable to stop scratching. Consult him immediately if your child is feverish or complains of neckache when the spots have scabbed over and he should be feeling better.

WHAT MIGHT THE DOCTOR DO?

- Your doctor will prescribe an anti-infective cream if any of the spots is infected.
- If itchiness is causing your child sleepless nights, your doctor may prescribe a sedative.

WHAT CAN I DO TO HELP?

- If your child is still in nappies, change them frequently and leave them off whenever possible to allow the spots to scab over.
- Cut your child's fingernails short and discourage him from scratching.

SEE ALSO
Blister, *page 41*
Itching, *page 35*

MEASLES

Measles is an infectious childhood disease, caused by a virus, which has become less common since routine immunization was introduced. It is very contagious and has an incubation period of between eight and 14 days. The first indication of measles is usually symptoms similar to those of the **common cold**, with a **fever** that becomes increasingly higher, and small, white spots form inside the mouth, on the lining of cheeks (Koplik's spots). Your child's eyes may also be red and sore. The initial symptoms are followed about three days later by small, brownish-red spots behind the ears; these spots merge together to form a rash over the face and torso.

IS IT SERIOUS?

Measles is a deeply unpleasant childhood illness but it is not normally serious. However, in rare cases your child may develop complications, such as infection of the middle ear, or pneumonia.

POSSIBLE SYMPTOMS

- Runny nose and dry cough.
- Headache.
- Fever, rising as high as 40°C (104°F).
- Small, white spots inside the mouth.
- Red, sore eyes, intolerant of bright light.
- Brownish-red rash of small spots, starting behind the ears and spreading to the torso.

SITES OF RASH

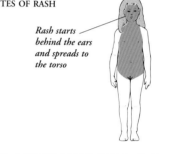

Rash starts behind the ears and spreads to the torso

WHAT SHOULD I DO FIRST?

1 Check your child's temperature. If he has a fever, try to bring it down with tepid sponging (see p. 26).

2 If your child's eyes are sore, bathe them with cool water.

3 Make sure he drinks plenty of fluids by offering small amounts regularly.

SHOULD I CONSULT THE DOCTOR?

Consult your doctor immediately if your child gets worse after seemingly recovering, or if he complains of **earache**.

WHAT MIGHT THE DOCTOR DO?

- Your doctor will advise you to keep your child in bed for as long as his temperature remains high. He will

examine your child's ears to check that there is no ear infection. If there is, he will prescribe a course of antibiotics.

- Your doctor may prescribe eye drops for your child's eyes if they are sore.

WHAT CAN I DO TO HELP?

- Don't send your child back to school until the rash has faded.
- Have any other children inoculated against measles. Immunization is advised at about 13 months of age.

SEE ALSO:
Common cold, *page 63*
Earache, *page 70*
Fever, *page 25*

MUMPS

Mumps is an infectious childhood disease, less common since routine immunization was introduced, and mostly affecting children over the age of two. It is caused by a virus and has an incubation period of 14 to 21 days. Your child will seem generally unwell for a day or two before the major symptoms appear. The salivary glands in front of and beneath the ears and chin swell up and there may be **fever.** The swelling can appear first on one side of the face, then the other, or on both sides at once, and cause pain when swallowing. He will complain of a dry mouth because the salivary glands have stopped producing saliva.

IS IT SERIOUS?

Mumps is a very mild disease. However, if before, during or after swelling, your child has a severe headache and a stiff neck, this could be encephalitis or **meningitis**, which are serious complications.

POSSIBLE SYMPTOMS

- Swollen, painful testes in boys, lower abdominal pain in girls.
- Swelling of the glands on either or both sides of the face just below the ears and beneath the chin.
- Pain when swallowing.
- Dry mouth.
- Headache.
- Fever.

AFFECTED
AREA

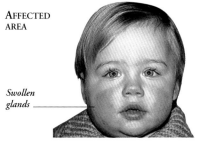

Swollen
glands

WHAT SHOULD I DO FIRST?

1 Check your child's temperature to see if he has a fever. If he has, try to bring it down with tepid sponging (see p. 26).

2 Liquidize his food if he is having difficulty eating and give him plenty to drink. Encourage him to rinse out his mouth to alleviate the dryness.

3 Put your child to bed with a hot-water bottle wrapped in a towel to hold against the affected side.

SHOULD I CONSULT THE DOCTOR?

Consult your doctor immediately to confirm the diagnosis, if your son's testes are painful or your daughter has abdominal pain. Consult him immediately if, after 10 days, his condition has worsened, and he has a headache and stiff neck.

WHAT MIGHT THE DOCTOR DO?

- There is no specific treatment for mumps. Your doctor will advise you to keep your child off school until five days after the swelling has gone down.
- If the testes are swollen, he will advise bed-rest until the swelling has subsided, and he will probably prescribe paracetamol for the pain of your son's testes or if your daughter has abdominal pain from swollen ovaries.

WHAT CAN I DO TO HELP?

Be inventive with liquid foods, such as egg-enriched milk shakes, soups and yoghurt, which slip down easily.

SEE ALSO:
Fever, *page 25*
Meningitis, *page 118*

GLANDULAR FEVER

Glandular fever, or infectious mono-nucleosis, is a viral infection that starts in much the same way as **influenza**, possibly with a rash similar to that of **rubella**. It is fairly common, affecting mostly teenagers and young adults; children can also contract it, but they tend to be less severely affected. There is no known cure for glandular fever and it has to run its course – usually, about a month. In reaction to the infection, the glands become swollen and the spleen may become enlarged. This does not in itself give rise to unpleasant symptoms, and the spleen will return to normal once the infection has gone.

POSSIBLE SYMPTOMS

- Swollen glands, most commonly in the neck, accompanied by a fever.
- Depression and lethargy.
- Rash which starts behind the ears, spreading to the forehead.
- Aches and pains.
- Runny nose.
- Sore throat.

AFFECTED AREA

Swollen glands

IS IT SERIOUS?

Glandular fever is not usually serious, but as so many of its symptoms are similar to those of other illnesses, you should consult your doctor for a diagnosis.

WHAT SHOULD I DO FIRST?

1 Many early symptoms are similar to those of other ailments, but be alerted if the neck glands are swollen and there is **fever***. Check his temperature regularly if his glands are swollen. If it remains high, give him a dose of liquid paracetamol.*

2 Keep him isolated until you have a confirmed diagnosis. The virus is infectious and is passed on by intimate contact, such as kissing.

SHOULD I CONSULT THE DOCTOR?

Consult your doctor immediately if you suspect your child is not just suffering from influenza or a **common cold**.

WHAT MIGHT THE DOCTOR DO?

Your doctor will take a blood sample. Glandular fever can be diagnosed with certainty only by finding antibodies in the blood. If the diagnosis is positive, you will be advised to keep your child indoors and to make sure he has plenty of rest; no further treatment is required.

WHAT CAN I DO TO HELP?

- Your child will not be able to return to school for at least a month. Don't send him back without your doctor's advice.
- If your child wants to stay in bed, let him. If he doesn't, keep him indoors until the fever subsides.
- If he has a temperature, offer him plenty of fluids to prevent dehydration.
- The virus may reappear during the two years after the first attack, so be alert for any recurrence of the symptoms and consult your doctor if you are worried.

SEE ALSO:
Common cold, *page 63*
Fever, *page 25*
Influenza, *page 87*
Rubella, *page 31*
Sore throat, *page 66*

RUBELLA

Rubella, or German measles, is a mild, infectious disease that is caused by a virus. It is contagious and has an incubation period of 14 to 21 days. The rash usually starts behind the ears before spreading to the forehead and the rest of the body. It looks more like a large patch of redness than a series of spots. The rash lasts about two to three days and is rarely accompanied by serious symptoms, just a mild fever and enlarged glands at the back of the neck. The main danger with rubella is not to your infected child but to any pregnant woman who may contract the disease from your child. Rubella can cause birth defects such as blindness and deafness.

IS IT SERIOUS?

This is not a serious childhood illness. However, you should keep your child in isolation for five days after the rash appears. Like other childhood infectious diseases, rubella carries a slight risk of encephalitis.

POSSIBLE SYMPTOMS

- Slightly raised temperature.
- Tiny pink or red spots, starting behind the ears and spreading to the forehead, then the rest of the body.
- Enlarged, swollen glands at the back of the neck.

SITE OF SWOLLEN GLANDS

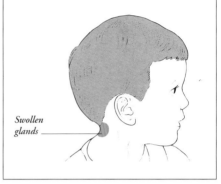

Swollen glands

WHAT SHOULD I DO FIRST?

1 Make sure that any woman who might be pregnant and has been in contact with your child is informed of your child's infection as quickly as possible.

2 Keep your child away from school and from public places where he is likely to come into contact with pregnant women and other children.

3 If your child's temperature rises above 38°C (100.4°F), give him a single dose of liquid paracetamol to bring it down.

4 If your child is feeling unwell, put him to bed.

SHOULD I CONSULT THE DOCTOR?

Consult your doctor by telephone to confirm that your child has rubella. Consult him immediately if your child complains of a stiff neck or a headache.

WHAT MIGHT THE DOCTOR DO?

There is no treatment for rubella, but your doctor will advise you to alert any women you know who might be pregnant, particularly those in the first four months of their pregnancy, if you haven't already done so.

WHAT CAN I DO TO HELP?

Make sure that all the children in your family are vaccinated against the disease.

AIDS

AIDS, or acquired immune deficiency syndrome, is a progressively debilitating condition caused by the human immuno-deficiency virus (HIV) that destroys the white blood cells in the body's immune system. In some cases HIV has been transferred via contaminated blood transfusions, but most HIV-infected children contract the virus from their mothers. However, not all HIV-positive mothers will transmit the virus to their fetus, and there are also some ways of reducing the risk before and around the time of the baby's delivery.

HIV infection produces few symptoms initially, but as it develops into AIDS, the immune system weakens, allowing diseases such as pneumonia to develop. Nearly all infected children will show symptoms before they are two years old, although some may not show any signs until they are more than five. To date, only a few children who are HIV-infected have made a full recovery, and without a major medical breakthrough, the outlook for HIV-positive people in general is bleak. Children with AIDS can expect to live for only a few years from the time when the symptoms first become apparent.

POSSIBLE SYMPTOMS
• Failure to thrive.
• Recurrent diarrhoea.
• Enlarged lymph nodes.
• Frequent infections.
• Attacks of pneumonia.
• Developmental delay.

SHOULD I CONSULT A DOCTOR?

If you suspect that your child has been infected with the HIV virus, seek your doctor's advice immediately. Children who are HIV-positive or who have developed AIDS need a high level of medical care.

WHAT CAN BE DONE?

• With your consent, a blood test will be performed to determine whether your baby is HIV-positive. Newborn babies of HIV-positive mothers can be difficult to diagnose because they do not show any symptoms of the virus, but their mother's antibodies may be present in their blood for at least a year.
• If your child is found to have the virus, your doctor may prescribe drugs to attack it and to slow the development and progress of the disease.
• Your doctor may give your child regular injections of gamma globulin and prescribe antibiotics to help prevent or fight any infections such as pneumonia.
• If you are HIV-positive, do not breast-feed your child as there is a small but important risk that you might transmit the virus to your baby via your milk.
• Your doctor will refer you to specialist organizations that can provide counselling and advice on how to manage the illness.

FOR HELP AND ADVICE CONTACT:
The Terrence Higgins Trust
52-54 Gray's Inn Road
London WC1X 8JU
0171 242 1010

CHAPTER

SKIN, HAIR AND NAILS

Because skin, hair and nails form the outer protective

covering for the body, they receive more than their

fair share of ailments and complaints. Those covered

in this chapter are among the most common you are

likely to encounter as your child grows up. In most

cases, minor ailments such as bruises, blisters and stings

are usually reasonably easily taken care of; but there are

other complaints such as burns, eczema and bites that

can be more serious. Each entry in the chapter takes

you through the realities as well as the possibilities and

provides practical assistance to see you through.

DIAGNOSIS GUIDE

Young children will get minor problems of the skin, hair, scalp and nails, but fortunately most are easily treated and cured. To use this section, look for the symptom most similar to the one that your child is suffering from or complaining of, then turn to the relevant entry. See also p.13 for a useful list of emergency symptoms.

YELLOW SCALES
on your baby's scalp *possibly*
Cradle cap, see p. 50

SMALL CRACKS
on the lips *possibly* **Chapping**,
see p. 45

FAINT RED RASH
over the neck, face, shoulders
and in the creases with a
flushed appearance *possibly*
Heat rash, see p. 44

ITCHY RED OR
GREY PATCH
that extends out in a ring
possibly **Ringworm**,
see p.56

WHITE, ITCHY LUMPS
in crops *possibly* **Hives**,
see p. 53

PIMPLY RED RASH
on the nappy area *possibly*
Nappy rash, see p. 49 or
Thrush, see p. 121

WHITE BLISTERED, ITCHY SKIN
between the toes *possibly*
Athlete's foot, see p.54

PAIN AND REDNESS
on the toenail *possibly*
Ingrowing toenail, see p. 59

ITCHY HEAD
with small eggs clinging to the
hair *possibly* **Lice**, see p. 57

TINY, ITCHY BLISTERS
around the lips *possibly* **Cold
sore**, see p. 48, or that ooze
and crust-over bright yellow
possibly **Impetigo**, see p. 55

PAINFUL RED LUMP
filled with pus *possibly* a
Boil, see p. 47

SMALL PUNCTURE MARK
possibly bee or wasp **Insect
stings**, see p. 40

FINE, SHORT, ITCHY
LINES IN THE SKIN
usually between the
fingers *possibly* **Scabies**
see p. 58

DRY, SCALY SKIN
with a red rash mainly on
the face, hands, wrists,
ankles and knees *possibly*
Eczema, see p. 51

NUMB, SWOLLEN
BLUE SKIN
that is itchy *possibly*
Chilblains, see p. 46

FLAT WHITE OR
BROWN LUMP
on the soles of the foot
possibly **Verruca**, see p. 60

34

ITCHING

Itching is nearly always a symptom of some underlying skin problem such as **eczema** or **ringworm**, the result of an infestation (**scabies**, fleas or worms), sensitivity to some foodstuff or drug, skin contact with an irritant (**hives**), or the result of an infectious disease such as **chickenpox**. From time to time nervous tension and worry can cause itching, and scratching can make the itchiness even worse.

IS IT SERIOUS?

Itching is rarely serious but it should not be ignored.

WHAT SHOULD I DO FIRST?

1 Try to determine the cause of the itching. The site may give you a clue. For example, itching around the anus and genitals could indicate worms or thrush, itchiness in the hair, ringworm, on the feet, athlete's foot or between the fingers, scabies.

2 Check any pets your child comes into contact with for fleas.

3 Check to see if your child has eaten any new foods recently.

4 Note whether your child is taking any new medicines.

5 Try soothing the itching with calamine lotion or give your child a cool bath with a handful of bicarbonate of soda dissolved in the water.

SHOULD I CONSULT THE DOCTOR?

Consult your doctor as soon as possible if you can find no apparent reason for the itching or if your child is having difficulty sleeping properly because of constant itchiness.

WHAT MIGHT THE DOCTOR DO?

• Your doctor will examine your child carefully to determine the cause of the itching. If the itching is a symptom of some other condition, your doctor will treat this accordingly. He may, for example, prescribe antihistamine tablets, liquid paracetamol or cream to curb the itching.
• If your child is having difficulty sleeping, your doctor may prescribe a mild sedative.

WHAT CAN I DO TO HELP?

• Dress your child in cotton underwear so that fabrics such as wool and nylon, which irritate, do not touch his skin.
• If you have recently changed your washing powder or fabric conditioner, change back to the old brand and see if the irritation subsides. Rinse clothes well.
• Use a mild soap and shampoo for your child.
• To stop your child scratching, put mittens on his hands whenever possible, and keep his nails short to prevent infection should he break the skin by scratching too hard.

SEE ALSO:
Athlete's foot, *page 54*
Chickenpox, *page 27*
Chilblains, *page 46*
Eczema, *page 51*
Hives, *page 53*
Ringworm, *page 56*
Scabies, *page 58*
Thrush, *page 121*

CUTS AND GRAZES

Small cuts and grazes can be treated at home, and should be cleaned up and possibly dressed to prevent germs causing infection. Dress with a piece of sterile gauze held in place with adhesive tape so that the air can get to the wound; plasters can also be used to dress a cut. If the cut is a deep one, a few stitches might be necessary, and if there is a lot of blood loss, shock might follow.

ARE THEY SERIOUS?

Cuts and grazes are not serious. However, if a cut is deep, there is a risk of infection.

WHAT SHOULD I DO FIRST?

If the wound is large and bleeding

1 Press firmly on the wound to compress the ends of the damaged blood vessels and raise the injured area above his heart.

2 Help him lie down with his head low and put a thin pad under his head. Keep the injured area raised and press on the wound for up to 10 minutes.

3 Cover the wound with a non-fluffy dressing larger than the wound itself, still keeping the injured area raised above the heart. Secure the dressing with a firmly-tied bandage. If blood seeps through, secure another dressing with a bandage on top. If necessary, support the wounded area in a sling. Call for an ambulance immediately.

If the wound is a small cut or graze

1 Sit your child down and gently wash the cut or graze with soap and water, making sure you remove all dirt or grit. If this causes a little fresh bleeding, press the wound with a clean pad.

2 Dress the wound with a plaster that has a pad large enough to cover it. Do not cover with cotton wool: fluffy materials stick to a wound and delay healing.

SHOULD I CONSULT THE DOCTOR?

Consult your doctor immediately or take your child to the nearest casualty department if the wound is large, if bleeding persists after 10 minutes of pressure, if the wound is very deep and bloody, if the wound is on the face, if the wound is gaping, if there is dirt or a foreign body in the wound that you can't get out, if the wound is deep but has only a small puncture hole in the skin or if your child was playing in an area where horses are kept and the wound has been contaminated by dirt or grit. Consult your doctor as soon as possible if, after a day or two, you notice any red streaks extending from the centre of the wound as this could be a sign of infection.

WHAT MIGHT THE DOCTOR DO?

• The doctor will clean the wound and stitch it, if necessary; any face wound will be stitched to minimize scarring.
• If the bleeding doesn't stop, a blood vessel may have been lacerated and this will be tied off under an anaesthetic.
• If there is a deep wound, or a wound contaminated with dirt, the doctor will give your child a tetanus injection if he has not had a booster.
• If there is any infection, the doctor will cover the area with an antibiotic dressing and he will probably also prescribe antibiotics.

WHAT CAN I DO TO HELP?

Change the dressing daily. Leave the dressing off at night as wounds heal more quickly if exposed to the air.

BITES

Most children love the company of animals, but because they are not always as gentle with them as they should be, bites can and do occur. The most common animal bites – from household pets such as dogs and cats – leave puncture marks; humans leave teeth marks. Insect bites leave a weal resembling **hives** – a white centre on a red base. They are extremely itchy, but the pain and localized reaction usually fade within three to four hours. The bites of the common flea, normally from a household pet, also leave itchy weals.

ARE THEY SERIOUS?

Animal, human and insect bites are rarely serious. If they are untreated, however, they could become infected.

WHAT SHOULD I DO FIRST?

1 Reassure your child and calm him down. If he has been bitten by a dog or a horse, for example, it is important that he does not remain afraid of these animals throughout his childhood. Try to persuade him that it is an isolated incident.

2 For animal and human bites, wash the wound with soap and water to remove any blood, saliva or dirt. Apply an antiseptic cream, then put a clean dressing over the wound.

3 For insect bites, apply calamine lotion to relieve the irritation.

SHOULD I CONSULT THE DOCTOR?

Consult your doctor as soon as possible to check that an animal or human bite is not infected or deep enough to carry the risk of tetanus. Consult your doctor immediately if the wound is bleeding heavily or if, after 12 hours, the area looks red and swollen.

WHAT MIGHT THE DOCTOR DO?

• Your child may need to be immunized against tetanus.
• If the wound is infected, your doctor will probably prescribe antibiotics.

WHAT CAN I DO TO HELP?

• You must emphasize to your child the need to treat animals carefully and not to tease them. In most cases, if a pet caused the injury, it will be an isolated incident and you should not need to get rid of the animal.
• If you are travelling abroad, be prepared for any problems by carrying a first-aid pack and updating tetanus boosters before you go.
• You will need to clean the carpet, curtains and furniture if you suspect that your child has been bitten by fleas. A special flea powder to dust furnishings is available from veterinary surgeons. Take your pet along to the vet for treatment too.
• If your child is being bitten by mosquitoes, apply an insect repellent to his skin or clothes, and put an incense stick in his room at night, or spray the room with an insect repellent.

SEE ALSO:
Hives, *page 53*

BRUISE

A bruise is a purplish-red stain in the skin, usually resulting from a blow or a knock that ruptures the small blood vessels near the skin's surface. Children with fair skin show a bruise more readily than children with olive skin. It usually takes 10–14 days for a bruise to disappear completely; as it fades, it changes colour to maroon, then green or yellow as the blood pigments break down and are reabsorbed by the body.

IS IT SERIOUS?

A bruise is rarely serious. If a bruise appears without any reason, this could relate to uncommon but serious conditions such as leukaemia and haemophilia.

POSSIBLE SYMPTOMS

• Purplish-red mark on the skin which fades to maroon and then green or yellow.
• Tenderness for a day or two.
• Swelling if the bruise is over a bone.

WHAT SHOULD I DO FIRST?

1 *A minor bruise needs no treatment at all, just a cuddle and reassurance if your child is upset.*

2 *If the bruise is large, apply a cold compress for half an hour or so. This will contain the bruising.*

SHOULD I CONSULT THE DOCTOR?

Consult your doctor immediately if pain on the site of the bruise gets worse after 24 hours: an underlying bone could be broken. Consult your doctor immediately if a bruise appears spontaneously with no apparent cause.

WHAT MIGHT THE DOCTOR DO?

• Your doctor will examine your child to determine if there is a **broken bone** and refer you to a hospital casualty department for treatment if necessary.
• Your doctor will refer you to a specialist clinic if your child suffers from recurrent bruising or bruises that appear spontaneously. This could indicate haemophilia or leukaemia.

SEE ALSO:
Broken bone, *page 110*

SPLINTER

A splinter is a tiny sliver of material that becomes embedded in or under the skin. It may be wood, metal, glass or a thorn.

IS IT SERIOUS?

A splinter is very rarely serious, although it can often be painful and uncomfortable.

It is therefore hardly ever necessary to get medical assistance; most splinters can be removed quite easily at home.

However, occasionally splinters can cause deep wounds. Such wounds can be serious, particularly if they do not bleed much, because they carry the risk of tetanus.

WHAT SHOULD I DO FIRST?

1 Find out from your child, if possible, what material is embedded in the skin. If it is glass, the entire surface of the splinter will be capable of cutting into your child's flesh, so don't try to remove it yourself; seek medical aid.

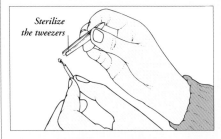

Sterilize the tweezers

2 If the splinter is not glass and the end is sticking out of the skin, remove it with tweezers. Sterilize them first by passing the ends through a flame.

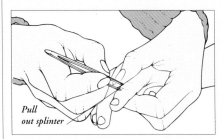

Pull out splinter

3 Allow the tweezers to cool, then distract your child so that he doesn't flinch too much as you gently pull out the splinter.

4 If the splinter is under the skin, sterilize a sharp needle with a flame or by standing it in some surgical spirit for a few minutes. Place a piece of ice over the splinter area so that the skin is lightly numbed, then use the sterile needle to break the skin's surface and expose the splinter. Once the end of the splinter is free, pull it out with a pair of sterilized tweezers.

5 Clean the area with soap and water and apply antiseptic cream. Don't put a plaster on unless your child asks for one.

6 If you experience any difficulty while trying to remove a splinter, abandon the attempt and obtain medical help.

SHOULD I CONSULT THE DOCTOR?

Consult your doctor immediately if the splinter is glass, if it is deep in the skin, or if it's contaminated with garden material (which increases the risk of tetanus). You should also contact your doctor if you cannot remove it easily yourself.

WHAT MIGHT THE DOCTOR DO?

• If the splinter is a piece of glass, or if it is deep in the skin, your doctor will remove it under a local anaesthetic.
• If there is any garden material in the wound, your doctor may give your child a tetanus booster injection.

INSECT STINGS

Most stings cause only local irritation and pain. In the rare cases where there is a severe allergic reaction to a sting, *anaphylactic shock* may develop. Bee and wasp stings make a small puncture hole in the skin; bees leave their stings behind but wasps rarely do.

ARE THEY SERIOUS?

A sting is rarely serious. However, if it causes an allergic reaction with severe swelling leading to loss of consciousness, if it is in the mouth or throat, or if your child is stung by a number of insects, then it should be treated as an emergency.

POSSIBLE SYMPTOMS

- Small puncture mark, with or without the sting left behind.
- Localized swelling and irritation.
- Breathing difficulties.
- Signs of shock – rapid pulse, clammy and pale skin, shortness of breath, sweating and faintness.

APPEARANCE OF A BEE STING

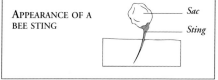

Sac

Sting

WHAT SHOULD I DO FIRST?

Keep him as calm and still as possible to slow down the rate the poison spreads.

If your child is stung by a bee or wasp

1 If the sting is still in the skin, scrape it off. Avoid squeezing the sac because this will force more poison into your child's body.

2 To reduce the pain and swelling, lay on a cold compress of diluted vinegar for wasp and bicarbonate of soda and water paste for bee stings. Don't rub the area.

If the sting is in the mouth or throat

1 If the sting is visible, remove it with tweezers. Avoid squeezing the sac. Give him cold water to drink or an ice cube to suck. If the sting is not visible, seek help.

2 If the area swells quickly, lay him down on his side and get medical help immediately.

SHOULD I CONSULT THE DOCTOR?

Take your child to the nearest casualty department if he has an allergic reaction or has been stung more than once by an insect. Consult your doctor immediately if he develops shock or breathing difficulties, if he has been stung in the throat or mouth and you can't remove the sting, or if the area is swelling.

WHAT MIGHT THE DOCTOR DO?

- The doctor or casualty department officer, if you go there, will treat your child for shock.
- If your child has suffered an allergic reaction, your doctor may prescribe antihistamine tablets or cream, depending on the severity. He may also give him a series of desensitizing injections to prevent the same reaction in future.
- Your doctor will remove the sting from your child's mouth if you've been unable to do so, and will control any swelling.

WHAT CAN I DO TO HELP?

- Make up an emergency pack of antihistamine medication if your child suffers an allergic reaction to insect stings. Carry it with you on holidays and outings.
- Keep an aerosol sting reliever with you on picnics and outings.

BLISTER

A blister is a fluid-filled bubble of skin that forms as a result of **burns** or friction, or as a result of exposure to extremes of temperature. Blisters vary in size, depending on the cause, and their purpose is to form a cushion to protect the new layer of skin growing underneath. The fluid is eventually reabsorbed by the body and the outer surface dries out and peels away, leaving the healed skin behind. If the blister is broken before healing has taken place, there is a risk of infection.

<table>
<tr><td>

POSSIBLE SYMPTOMS

• Raised surface of the skin, filled with fluid, which may be as large as several centimetres across.

</td></tr>
</table>

IS IT SERIOUS?

A blister is not usually serious.

WHAT SHOULD I DO FIRST?

1 Don't prick a blister that has formed as a result of friction, burning or extremes of temperature; leave it intact.

2 Protect blisters where friction may cause them to burst. For example, if the blister is a result of ill-fitting shoes or wearing shoes without socks, change your child's shoes for the time being, put two pairs of socks on your child, or use special sponge pads or corn plasters to protect the blister.

3 If the blister bursts, keep it clean and dry and cover it with a gauze dressing.

SHOULD I CONSULT THE DOCTOR?

Consult your doctor as soon as possible if the blister is large or the result of a scald or **sunburn**. Consult your doctor as soon as possible if the area becomes infected, that is, if the blister becomes pus-filled, if red streaks extend outwards from it, if the skin surrounding it becomes red, tender or swollen, or if your child complains of pain.

WHAT MIGHT THE DOCTOR DO?

• If the blister is large, it may require bursting. Your doctor will do this.
• If the blister is infected, your doctor will prescribe antibiotics.

SEE ALSO:
Burn, *page 42*
Cold sore, *page 48*
Sunburn, *page 43*

BURN

A burn is an injury to the skin following exposure to heat such as fire or electric current. The severity will depend on the situation and the cause. In a *superficial burn* there may be just a reddened patch of skin or a **blister**; in a *deep burn,* layers of skin may actually be removed.

POSSIBLE SYMPTOMS
- Raw, red areas.
- Fluid-filled blisters.
- Small blackened area after an electric current has touched the skin.

IS IT SERIOUS?

Apart from very superficial ones, all burns should be treated seriously, but electrical burns should be treated with particular caution because they may be deep but appear minor. Only small, superficial burns should be treated at home, for no matter how minor a burn may seem to be, there will always be some damage to the underlying tissue (in deep burns there may not always be pain, because nerve endings have been damaged). All burns ooze a colourless liquid (*serum*), and if too much is lost, your child could go into shock.

WHAT SHOULD I DO FIRST?

For small, superficial burns

1 Cool the affected area by placing under cold running water for 10–15 minutes.

2 Cover with a sterile dressing extended beyond the injured area. Don't apply creams or lotions, certainly not butter or fat. Give your child liquid paracetamol to relieve the pain.

3 Raise the affected part slightly so that blood flow to the area is slowed down. This will help to ease the pain.

For deep or electrical burns

1 If the burns were caused by liquids, use a cloth to prevent them from getting on to your skin, and take off your child's clothing. They will continue to burn him until they are removed. Do not remove any clothing that is sticking to the skin.

2 If your child has suffered an electric shock, first break his contact with the electricity by turning off the current or knocking him away with a non-conducting material, such as wood.

3 Cool the affected area by running cold water over it for as long as possible. If it covers a large area, put him into a cool bath.

4 Cover the affected area with a sterile dressing. Don't apply any creams or lotions, certainly not butter or fat.

5 To prevent shock, lay your child down with his legs raised and supported and his head turned to one side. Wrap him in a clean sheet to reduce the risk of infection.

SHOULD I CONSULT THE DOCTOR?

Only small, superficial burns should be treated at home; consult your doctor immediately for all other types. Consult your doctor if a superficial burn does not heal in a week, or if the area becomes red and swollen and pus forms.

WHAT MIGHT THE DOCTOR DO?

If the burn is infected, your doctor will cover the area with an antibiotic dressing.

SEE ALSO:
Blister, *page 41*

SUNBURN

Sunburn is inflammation of the skin caused by excessive exposure to the ultra-violet rays in sunlight. It is always due to misjudgement or carelessness on the part of the parent. The best cure is prevention. Even adults should give all but deep olive or black skins a chance to gradually acclimatize to the sun. It is necessary to be strict with children who may not appreciate the dangers. Your child's sunburn can result in tender and damaged skin that may blister or peel off. Even in mild sunshine, the effects of the sun can be increased if you are near water, snow or sand, where the rays are reflected off the bright surface.

POSSIBLE SYMPTOMS

- Red, hot, tender skin.
- Blisters.
- Itchiness prior to peeling skin.

IS IT SERIOUS?

Sunburn can be very serious if a large area of the skin is burned. The skin may lose its ability to regulate body temperature effectively so that your child's temperature soars and heatstroke results. There is also a major long-term risk of skin cancer.

WHAT SHOULD I DO FIRST?

1 *Apply a soothing lotion such as calamine to any tight, red skin to cool it down and reduce the irritation.*

2 *When you're inside, don't put any clothing on the sunburned areas; leave them exposed to the air. Cover sunburned areas when you are outside.*

3 *If blisters appear and your child complains of pain, give him paracetamol. Take his temperature to see if he has a fever. If it is over 39°C (102.2°F), consult your doctor and try to reduce with tepid sponging (see p. 26).*

4 *Keep your child out of direct sunlight for at least 48 hours.*

SHOULD I CONSULT THE DOCTOR?

Consult your doctor if blisters form on your child's sunburned skin and he is feverish. Consult your doctor immediately if your child has a fever but his skin is dry and he seems confused and drowsy; it could be heatstroke, which should be treated as an emergency.

WHAT MIGHT THE DOCTOR DO?

- In a mild case of sunburn, your doctor may prescribe a soothing cream.
- If blisters have formed and your child is feverish, your doctor may prescribe an anti-inflammatory cream to help the skin to heal more quickly.
- If your child is suffering from heatstroke, he will treat this accordingly.

WHAT CAN I DO TO HELP?

- Draw the sheets on your child's bed tightly so that nothing scratches his tender skin.
- To prevent sunburn, keep all but the toughest parts of your child's skin covered up for the first few days of bright sunlight. From then on, apply a total sunblock lotion to all the exposed parts of his body and protect the nape of his neck with a wide-brimmed hat.
- Remember to apply the sunblock again after your child has been swimming.
- Increase exposure to sun by 10-minute increments only each day.
- Keep a check on your child's skin and if it is starting to burn, cover him up immediately.

HEAT RASH

Heat rash is a faint red rash in the areas of the body where the sweat glands are most numerous – on the face, neck and shoulders, and in the skin creases, such as the elbows, groin and behind the knees. It is quite common in babies because their sweat glands are still primitive and not efficient at regulating body temperature. Heat rash is not due to exposure to sunlight, but arises when the body becomes overheated and the skin responds with excessive production of sweat.

IS IT SERIOUS?

Heat rash is never serious.

POSSIBLE SYMPTOMS

AREAS AFFECTED

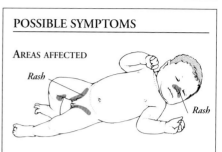

Rash

Rash

• Faint red rash over the face, neck, shoulders and in the creases, such as the elbows, groin and knees.
• Flushed and hot appearance.

WHAT SHOULD I DO FIRST?

1 Check your baby's clothing. He may be wearing too many clothes for the air temperature.

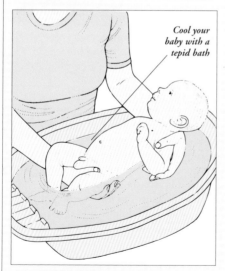

Cool your baby with a tepid bath

2 Undress your baby and bathe him in tepid water. Gently pat him dry to remove most of the moisture. Allow the rest to evaporate – this will cool his skin down.

SHOULD I CONSULT THE DOCTOR?

There is no need to consult the doctor for a heat rash. Consult your doctor as soon as possible if the rash does not disappear 12 hours after the baby has cooled down.

WHAT MIGHT THE DOCTOR DO?

Your doctor will examine your baby to exclude any other reason for the rash, and will probably advise you to dress your baby in natural fibres, which do not trap the sweat.

WHAT CAN I DO TO HELP?

• Check that the temperature in your baby's room is not too high. Keep the air flowing by opening a window slightly.
• Don't overdress your child when the weather is hot.
• Don't put wool or synthetic fibres directly against your baby's skin. Dress him in a cotton vest first.

CHAPPING

Chaps are small cracks in the skin that can be painful if they are deep. In nearly all cases, chapping is preceded by drying out of the skin due to its exposure to cold air or to hot, dry air. Chapping is therefore most common in exposed parts of the body such as on the lips, fingers, hands and ears.

POSSIBLE SYMPTOMS

- Small cracks in the skin, most commonly on the lips, fingers, hands and ears.
- Bleeding, if the cracks are deep.

IS IT SERIOUS?

Chapping is not serious.

WHAT SHOULD I DO FIRST?

1 Keep your child's skin well moisturized with cream.

2 Keep your child warm in cold weather, particularly his hands and ears.

3 If your child has dry lips, put lip salve or Vaseline on regularly throughout the day.

4 If the chap cracks, place a piece of surgical tape or adhesive tape over it, where possible, for about 12 hours, to stop it drying out and cracking even more. Do not do this to a young baby – he could swallow the tape.

SHOULD I CONSULT THE DOCTOR?

Consult your doctor as soon as possible if the chaps fail to heal properly or if they become infected.

WHAT MIGHT THE DOCTOR DO?

- Your doctor may prescribe an emollient cream to keep the skin moist.
- If there is an infection, your doctor will prescribe antibiotics.

WHAT CAN I DO TO HELP?

Don't wash your child with soap too often during cold weather. Soap defats the skin and makes it rough. An emollient cream or baby lotion can be used instead of soap to clean the skin.

SEE ALSO:
Chilblains, *page 46*

CHILBLAINS

Chilblains are areas of red, itchy skin that are the result of a hypersensitivity to cold. When the skin of a cold-sensitive child is exposed to cold and damp, the blood vessels beneath the skin close up to conserve heat, causing the skin to become numb and pale. When the blood vessels dilate again with warmth, the skin becomes red and itchy. Chilblains usually appear on the ankles, hands and feet, and on the back of the legs.

ARE THEY SERIOUS?

Chilblains are not serious, but they can be very irritating.

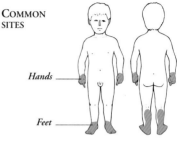

POSSIBLE SYMPTOMS

• Pale, numb skin, particularly on the hands and feet.

COMMON SITES

Hands

Feet

• Red, swollen and itchy skin when the area warms up.

WHAT SHOULD I DO FIRST?

1 If your child has been out in the cold without sufficient warm clothing and then complains of itchiness, dust the skin with talcum powder or cornflour to ease the irritation.

2 Stop your child from breaking the skin of the affected areas by covering them with clothing or putting mittens on him.

SHOULD I CONSULT THE DOCTOR?

Consult your doctor as soon as possible if the chilblains give your child a great deal of discomfort.

WHAT MIGHT THE DOCTOR DO?

Your doctor may prescribe a vasodilator cream to improve circulation.

WHAT CAN I DO TO HELP?

• Keep all the susceptible parts on your child's body covered up and warm in damp and cold weather.
• Put thermal insoles in your child's shoes to keep his feet warm.

SEE ALSO
Itching, *page 35*

BOIL

A boil is a large, tender, red lump that results when a hair follicle becomes infected with bacteria (*staphylococci*). The pus-filled lump gradually comes to a head and bursts after about two or three days, or it may heal on its own without bursting and slowly disappear. Because the hair follicles are so close together, the bacteria can infect a wide area, causing more boils to occur. This is most likely to happen on the face. The boils usually appear on areas where there are pressure points, such as where a collar rubs, or on the buttocks.

IS IT SERIOUS?

Although unsightly, a boil is not serious. It can, however, be painful, especially if it develops over a bony area such as the jaw, where the skin is stretched tight.

POSSIBLE SYMPTOMS

- Large, painful, red lump.
- Increasing tenderness and throbbing as pus builds up inside the lump. After a day or two, the red lump forms a white or yellow pus-filled centre, which may or may not burst.

CROSS–SECTION OF SKIN

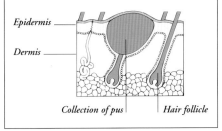

Epidermis

Dermis

Collection of pus   *Hair follicle*

WHAT SHOULD I DO FIRST?

1 Wash the skin with surgical spirit or 5ml (1 teaspoonful) of salt in a glass of warm water to prevent the infection from spreading. Then put a sterile gauze dressing over the boil.

2 Do not squeeze the boil, even when it comes to a head. Squeezing will spread the infection to the surrounding area.

SHOULD I CONSULT THE DOCTOR?

Consult your doctor as soon as possible if the boil does not come to a head within five days, or is causing a lot of pain. Consult him as soon as possible if red streaks spread from the centre; it could mean that the infection is spreading.

WHAT MIGHT THE DOCTOR DO?

- Your doctor will examine the boil and the surrounding area. If he can feel pus under the skin, he will probably lance it and drain the pus, reducing the pain.

- If there is an infection, or if your child has had a number of boils over the previous months, he may prescribe an anti-infective cream to treat the skin's surface, or antibiotic tablets to prevent the internal spread of the infection.
- If there are crops of boils, your doctor may prescribe a special antiseptic to put in the bath water.
- If the boils are recurrent, your child will be referred to a dermatologist to find out the underlying cause.

WHAT CAN I DO TO HELP?

- Once the boil has burst, keep covered to stop your child from scratching the area.
- If the boil is in a place where clothing might rub it, put a thick pad over the dressing to prevent any friction.
- If his boil is on the buttocks and he is still in nappies, leave them off as much as possible and use an antiseptic cream around the site.

COLD SORE

Cold sores are tiny **blisters** that form mostly around the nostrils and lips but sometimes also elsewhere on the face. The blisters break open and weep before they crust over and disappear. Cold sores are caused by a virus (*Herpes simplex*) that lives permanently in the nerve endings of some adults and children. A rise in skin temperature – perhaps caused by a cold, or by going out in the sun – activates the virus. The first attack may take the form of painful **mouth ulcers**. Subsequent attacks take the form of skin blisters. Most cold sores last about 10–14 days.

POSSIBLE SYMPTOMS

- Raised red area, usually around the nostrils and lips, which tingles and feels itchy. Tiny blisters then form on the spot.
- Weeping blisters, which then crust over.

IS IT SERIOUS?

Cold sores are not serious unless they occur near the eye, where they may rarely cause an ulcer to form on the front of the eyeball.

WHAT SHOULD I DO FIRST?

1 Once blisters have formed, stop your child from touching the area. Keep his hands clean.

2 Apply surgical spirit to the cold sores to dry them up, or smear a soothing cream such as Vaseline on to them to keep them moist while the virus runs its course. One or the other treatment may give your child some relief.

SHOULD I CONSULT THE DOCTOR?

Consult your doctor as soon as possible if a cold sore is near your child's eye. Consult your doctor as soon as possible if the cold sores become redder and develop pus-filled centres; they will have become infected with bacteria. Ask your doctor's advice if your child suffers from recurrent cold sores.

WHAT MIGHT THE DOCTOR DO?

- If the cold sores are infected, your doctor will prescribe an antibiotic ointment that lubricates the area and treats the infection.
- Your doctor may prescribe an antiviral cream to spread over the affected area regularly to contain the attack. He may prescribe antiviral tablets, if attacks are frequent.

WHAT CAN I DO TO HELP?

- Make sure that your child uses his own towel and facecloth.
- Don't let your child kiss anyone, especially other children. The virus can be transmitted this way.
- If your child tends to develop cold sores after exposure to sunlight, smear a sunblock on his lips or nose when he plays out in the sun.

SEE ALSO
Blister, *page 41*
Mouth ulcer, *page 81*
Sunburn, *page 43*

NAPPY RASH

Nappy rash is a skin condition that affects the area normally covered by a baby's nappy, and can occur whether the nappies used are fabric or disposable.

There are several causes of nappy rash, but it is most commonly caused by urine and stools being left in contact with the skin for too long. Bottle-fed babies are more likely to suffer from this form of nappy rash than breastfed ones.

Nappy rash can also be caused by inadequate drying after bathing your baby. In such cases the nappy rash is usually confined to the skin creases at the top of the thighs. If the rash covers most of the nappy area, and you use fabric nappies, it may be due to an allergic reaction to chemicals in the washing powder used to wash them, or to fabric conditioner. This reaction is an early sign of a form of **eczema** known as atopic eczema.

POSSIBLE SYMPTOMS

- Redness over nappy area.
- Redness that starts around the genitals and is accompanied by a strong smell of ammonia.
- Tight, papery skin with inflamed spots that have pus-filled centres.
- Redness that starts around the anus and moves over the buttocks and on to the thighs.

A rash that starts around the anus and moves over the buttocks and on to the thighs may not be nappy rash at all but a **thrush** infection.

IS IT SERIOUS?

Nappy rash is not serious and can be easily prevented and treated at home.

WHAT SHOULD I DO FIRST?

1 When you notice redness on your baby's bottom, wash it with warm water and dry thoroughly. Apply barrier cream to prevent skin irritation. If he wears disposable nappies use only a small amount.

2 Change nappies and wash your baby's bottom at least every two to three hours and as soon as he's had a bowel motion. Leave off the nappy whenever possible.

3 Use one-way disposable nappy liners next to his skin, as these are designed to let urine pass through to the nappy while remaining dry. Don't use talcum powder around his genitals. It irritates the skin.

4 Check inside his mouth. If there are white patches, try to wipe them off. If they leave raw, red patches, your baby has oral thrush, which may have caused the rash.

SHOULD I CONSULT THE DOCTOR?

Consult the doctor if these measures fail to clear the rash within a few days, or if you think your baby has thrush.

WHAT MIGHT THE DOCTOR DO?

- If the nappy rash has become infected, your doctor may prescribe antibiotics.
- If your baby has signs of eczema, he may advise you to change your brand of washing powder or conditioner. He may prescribe a cortisone ointment to be used sparingly.
- If the nappy rash is caused by thrush, your doctor will prescribe an anti-fungal cream.

SEE ALSO

Eczema, *page 51*
Thrush, *page 121*

CRADLE CAP

Cradle cap is a thick yellow encrustation on the scalp. It occurs mainly in babies, though children up to the age of three can have cradle cap. The yellow scales appear in small patches or can cover the entire scalp. Cradle cap is not due to poor hygiene. Babies who suffer from it probably just have greasier scalps.

POSSIBLE SYMPTOM

• Thick, yellowish scales over part or all of the scalp.

IS IT SERIOUS?

Cradle cap may appear unsightly, but it is quite harmless unless it is accompanied by red, scaly areas elsewhere on your baby's body, in which case your baby may have seborrhoeic **eczema.**

WHAT SHOULD I DO FIRST?

1 Do not try to remove the scales with your fingers. If they won't brush out, they must be loosened first.

2 Smear a little baby oil or Vaseline on to your baby's scalp and leave overnight. This makes the scales soft and loose and they will wash away when you shampoo the next day.

3 Do not use anti-dandruff shampoos without consulting your doctor.

SHOULD I CONSULT THE DOCTOR?

Consult your doctor if you are worried about the condition or if your baby has any red, scaly areas elsewhere.

WHAT MIGHT THE DOCTOR DO?

Your doctor or health visitor will prescribe a special shampoo to prevent the scales from forming and give you advice on brushing and other home treatments that help prevent cradle cap.

WHAT CAN I DO TO HELP?

• You can prevent scales from building up by brushing through your baby's hair daily, even if there is very little of it, with a soft-bristled brush.

• Never rub the scalp very hard when washing your child's hair. Shampoos remove dirt within seconds, so you only need to bring the shampoo to a lather and then rinse it off thoroughly.

• If the cradle cap becomes quite hard and thick, you may have to continue the baby oil or Vaseline treatment over a 10-day period to loosen all the encrustations.

SEE ALSO
Eczema, *page 51*

ECZEMA

Eczema is an allergic skin condition which produces an extremely itchy, dry, scaly, red rash on the face, neck and hands, and in the creases of the limbs.

The most common form of eczema in children is *atopic eczema*, which usually develops when a baby is about two to three months old, or at around the age of four to five months, when solid foods are first introduced into his diet. Certain foods, most commonly dairy products, eggs and wheat, and skin irritants such as pet fur, wool or washing powders, are among the main causes. An attack of eczema can also be triggered by stress or an emotional upset of any kind. It is quite common for eczema to be followed by other allergic complaints such as **hayfever** and penicillin sensitivity. It is also quite common for a child with eczema to suffer from **asthma**. Although most children grow out of eczema by the age of three, the associated allergic conditions may remain.

POSSIBLE SYMPTOMS

- Dry, red scaly skin which is extremely itchy. The rash usually starts off as minute pearly blisters beneath the skin's surface.
- Sleeplessness if the itchiness is very bad.

Another form of eczema, known as *seborrhoeic eczema*, occurs where the sebaceous glands are numerous, most commonly on the scalps of young babies (**cradle cap**), on the eyelashes and eyelids, in the external ear canal (**otitis externa**) and in the greasy areas around the nostrils, ears and groin. Seborrhoeic eczema is not as itchy as atopic eczema and responds well to treatment.

IS IT SERIOUS?

Eczema is not serious, although it can be very irritating.

WHAT SHOULD I DO FIRST?

1 If your child is scratching, inspect his neck, scalp, face, hands and the creases of his elbows, knees and groin for any rash.

2 Keep his fingernails short to minimize the possibility of breaking the skin. If the skin becomes broken, put mittens or gloves on him to prevent him from scratching the affected area.

3 If you've just started weaning your breastfed child, return to breast feeds until you see your doctor. If you have been using formula milk, return to that.

4 Apply an oily calamine lotion to ease irritation and soothe the skin. Don't apply any astringent lotions.

5 Stop washing your child with soap and water; it defats the skin. Use cleansing creams instead.

6 Put bath oil in his bath water to soothe the skin.

SHOULD I CONSULT THE DOCTOR?

Consult your doctor as soon as possible if you suspect your child may have eczema.

Continued on next page

ECZEMA: CONTINUED

WHAT MIGHT THE DOCTOR DO?

• Your doctor will question you on your family's medical history, and in particular whether anyone related to you or your partner has ever suffered from eczema-related conditions, such as asthma or hayfever.

• He will ask you about any changes in your child's diet, whether you have recently changed washing powders, whether you have just brought a pet into the house and whether your child wears natural or synthetic fibres.

• If you have just started weaning your baby from the breast or bottle, your doctor may recommend that you avoid dairy products and continue with breastfeeding or formula milk, or recommend soya milk instead.

• Your doctor may prescribe an anti-inflammatory skin cream to reduce redness, scaliness and itchiness. In severe cases, very weak steroid creams may be prescribed. These should be used sparingly. He may also recommend emollient creams or ointments.

• Your doctor may prescribe anti-histamine medication to help your child to sleep if the itching is keeping him awake at night.

• If your child's skin has become infected through scratching, your doctor may prescribe antibiotics.

• He will advise you to add bath oil to your child's bath water and to stop using soap as this can be an irritant. The oil will help to keep your child's skin supple and moisturized.

WHAT CAN I DO TO HELP?

• Continue to use an emollient cream whenever your child washes. This will keep his skin soft, prevent it from drying out and will damp down the itchiness as well.

• Underplay the condition in front of your child. Your anxiety can make the condition worse.

• Keep your child's fingernails short and put gloves or mittens on his hands at night so that scratching doesn't cause the skin to break and become infected.

• Make sure all of your child's clothes, and anything else that comes next to his skin, are rinsed thoroughly to remove all traces of any powders and fabric conditioners that could irritate his skin.

• You may need to consider giving your family pet away if the reaction is found to be caused by pet fur.

• Dress your child with cotton next to his skin at all times.

• Don't eliminate any foods from your child's diet without your doctor's supervision.

• Remove as many irritants from your child's environment as possible. For example, feather and down pillows can be a source of irritation.

SEE ALSO:

Asthma, *page 90*
Cradle cap, *page 50*
Hayfever, *page 89*
Itching, *page 35*
Nappy rash, *page 49*
Otitis externa, *page 71*

HIVES

Hives, urticaria, or nettle rash, is a skin condition. The rash that results is easy to recognize: the skin erupts into white lumps on a red base, known as weals. The weals can be as small as pimples, or be centimetres across. Hives can be caused by skin contact with an allergen, such as primulas, or it can result from eating certain foods, such as strawberries and shellfish, or from taking certain drugs, particularly penicillin and aspirin. Hives is common after a nettle sting. Each crop of weals is very itchy and lasts up to an hour. It then disappears, to be replaced by more weals elsewhere.

IS IT SERIOUS?

Hives is not serious, but if it appears on the face, especially in or around the mouth, and is accompanied by swelling, you should get medical assistance immediately. This allergic reaction is known as *angioneurotic oedema*, and if the swelling spreads to the tongue or the throat, it can cause severe breathing problems.

POSSIBLE SYMPTOMS

- White lumps on a red base.
- Extremely itchy rash.
- Weals which disappear within an hour or so to be replaced elsewhere by other weals.
- Swelling on the face.

CLASSIC APPEARANCE OF RASH

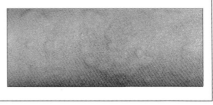

WHAT SHOULD I DO FIRST?

1 Apply calamine lotion to the weals to soothe the skin.

2 Give your child a warm bath to relieve itching.

SHOULD I CONSULT THE DOCTOR?

Consult your doctor immediately if hives on your child's face causes swelling, particularly in and around the mouth. Consult your doctor as soon as possible if the weals have not gone after several days, or if your child is miserable with the itchiness.

WHAT MIGHT THE DOCTOR DO?

- Your doctor may prescribe antihistamine tablets or medicine to relieve the itchiness of your child's skin.
- Your doctor may give your child an injection of adrenalin if the swelling is causing breathing problems.

WHAT CAN I DO TO HELP?

If your child has frequent attacks, make a note of any new foods he might have eaten. Provided it is not an essential food for a growing child, you can exclude it for a week or two, then reintroduce it and watch for a reaction.

SEE ALSO:
Itching, *page 35*

ATHLETE'S FOOT

This is a fungal infection that affects the soft area between and underneath the toes. In an advanced stage, it also affects the nails. It is contagious and is usually picked up by walking barefoot in communal areas, such as shower rooms, gymnasiums and swimming pools, where infected feet have been. The infection is aggravated by sweaty feet because the fungus, *tinea*, which also causes **ringworm** elsewhere on the body, thrives in warm, moist conditions.

IS IT SERIOUS?

Athlete's foot is a common condition, requiring only simple treatment and good hygiene to cure it. However, as it is contagious, you should act quickly so that the infection is not spread.

POSSIBLE SYMPTOMS

- White, blistered skin between and underneath the toes. The area is itchy and, when scratched, splits and leaves raw, red skin underneath.
- Dry, peeling skin.
- Thick, yellow toenails.

POSSIBLE SITES OF BLISTERED SKIN

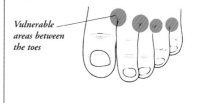

Vulnerable areas between the toes

WHAT SHOULD I DO FIRST?

1 If your child has itchy feet, carefully check the area between the toes and underneath them for any white blisters and redness.

2 Check underneath the foot for blisters and cracking.

3 Check the condition of your child's toenails.

4 Buy an antifungal foot powder or cream from your chemist, and, after washing and drying the feet thoroughly, apply the treatment, following the manufacturer's instructions.

5 Emphasize to your child that he must not go barefoot until the condition has cleared up.

6 Keep your child's towel and bath mat separate from those of the rest of the family and wash them every day.

SHOULD I CONSULT THE DOCTOR?

Consult your doctor as soon as possible if the underside of the foot is already affected, or if the nails are distorted or yellowing. Consult your doctor if the self-help measures fail to improve the condition within two or three weeks.

WHAT MIGHT THE DOCTOR DO?

- If the fungus has affected the toenails, your doctor will prescribe an antifungal medication that may need to be taken for as long as nine months.
- If your self-help measures failed, your doctor will prescribe another antifungal powder or cream.

WHAT CAN I DO TO HELP?

- Make sure your child has clean socks every day, preferably cotton or wool.
- Rotate your child's shoes.

IMPETIGO

Impetigo is a bacterial skin infection that is most often seen around the lips, nose and ears. It is caused by very common skin organisms (*staphylococcus* and *streptococcus*), which are carried in the nose and on the skin. The rash starts as small **blisters**, which break and then crust over to become yellow-brown scabs. The condition is most often seen in school-age children and is very contagious.

IS IT SERIOUS?

Impetigo rarely has serious effects, but because it is highly contagious, it should be treated immediately.

POSSIBLE SYMPTOM

• Tiny blisters around the nose and mouth or ears, which ooze and harden to form crusty, yellow-brown scabs.

WHAT SHOULD I DO FIRST?

1 If the rash on your child's face starts to weep, stop him from touching it. Gently wash away any crusts with warm water and pat his face dry with a paper towel. Make sure that your child's facecloth and towel are kept separate from those of the rest of the family to avoid spreading the infection.

2 Keep your child away from school until you have visited the doctor and confirmed the diagnosis.

SHOULD I CONSULT THE DOCTOR?

Consult your doctor as soon as possible if you suspect impetigo.

WHAT MIGHT THE DOCTOR DO?

• Your doctor will prescribe an anti-biotic cream which should clear up the impetigo within five days.
• Your doctor might also prescribe a course of antibiotics to be taken by mouth to eradicate the infection from your child's body, or a nasal cream to prevent the infection being spread to other parts of the body.

WHAT CAN I DO TO HELP?

• Before applying the ointment, wash away any yellow crusts with warm water and pat dry with a paper towel.
• Be meticulous about hygiene. Wash your hands before and after administering the treatment, and encourage your child to keep his hands away from his face. Keep his fingernails short to reduce the risk of spreading the infection to other parts of the body.
• Be very strict with your child if he sucks his thumb, bites his nails or picks his nose. This can spread the infection.
• When the infection has cleared, keep the area moist with emollient cream.

SEE ALSO
Blister, *page 41*

Ringworm

Ringworm is a fungal infection of the skin and hair that shows itself as bald patches in the hair, and as round, reddish or grey scaly patches on the skin. As the infection spreads, the edges of the ring remain scaly, and the centre begins to look more like normal skin. Ringworm is usually contracted from animals, such as a household pet, or from other infected humans.

POSSIBLE SYMPTOMS
• Red or grey scaly rings on any part of the body, particularly warm, moist areas, and on the scalp, where they produce bald patches.   • Itchiness in the ringed areas.

IS IT SERIOUS?

Although not a serious disorder, ringworm is unattractive and irritating. Ringworm is also very contagious and must therefore be treated promptly.

WHAT SHOULD I DO FIRST?

1 If your child is scratching, check all over his body for the distinctive rings of ringworm.

2 Do not try to treat it yourself. Wash your hands after examining your child. Discourage him from touching the infected areas.

3 Keep your child away from school until you have visited the doctor.

SHOULD I CONSULT THE DOCTOR?

Consult your doctor as soon as possible as ringworm is contagious as well as irritating for your child.

WHAT MIGHT THE DOCTOR DO?

Your doctor will prescribe an antifungal cream for the skin and antibiotic tablets for the scalp. The tablets will have to be taken for at least four weeks.

WHAT CAN I DO TO HELP?

• Throw out any brushes, combs or headgear your child may have used while infected. Disinfectant will not destroy the fungus.
• Keep your child's facecloth and towel separate from those of the rest of the family to avoid spreading the infection through the household.
• Always make sure that you and your child wash your hands thoroughly both before and after touching the affected areas.
• If you think that your pet is a possible source of ringworm, you should take it to the vet for treatment as soon as possible.
• Ringworm on the skin clears up quickly, but treatment of the scalp could take a couple of weeks or more. Get your child some form of headgear to hide the bald patches if he is bothered by them.

SEE ALSO
Itching, *page 35*

LICE (NITS)

The head louse is a tiny insect that infests the hair on the human head. The adult louse lays its eggs (nits) at the root of the hair, to which they become firmly attached. This distinguishes them from dandruff, which can be flaked off easily with a fingernail. The eggs hatch after two weeks and the lice bite the scalp to get blood. Your child's head will be itchy where the lice bite, particularly after strenuous exercise when he is hot. Your child can become infested by contact with another infested child or adult.

ARE THEY SERIOUS?

Lice and nits are irritating, but they can be easily eradicated and are not serious.

POSSIBLE SYMPTOMS

• Itchy scalp, particularly when the head is hot.

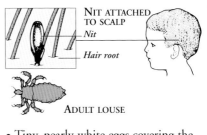

NIT ATTACHED TO SCALP
Nit
Hair root
ADULT LOUSE

• Tiny, pearly-white eggs covering the roots of the hair.

WHAT SHOULD I DO FIRST?

1 If your child scratches, inspect the roots of the hair for nits.

2 If you find them, keep your child away from school until you have administered the treatment recommended by schools (see below). You should inform the headteacher of the outbreak so that he can inform the health authorities.

3 First wash the hair, then soak the hair in plenty of conditioner and comb through with a nit comb.

4 If you find full-size lice or nits, repeat this process four times over the next two weeks.

5 Examine the heads of the rest of your family for nits, and treat in the same way. If anyone in your family has been in contact with someone who has lice, it is quite likely that the insects have transferred from one head to another.

SHOULD I CONSULT THE DOCTOR?

Consult your doctor before treating your child if he is less than two years old or has allergies. Consult him as soon as possible if the treatment doesn't work or if you are not sure your child has head lice.

WHAT MIGHT THE DOCTOR DO?

• Your doctor will question you about the self-help treatment you have used.
• He will probably report the outbreak to the health authorities; lice infestation is considered a public health hazard.

WHAT CAN I DO TO HELP?

• Clean your child's headgear, brush or combs thoroughly.
• If your child starts scratching again, repeat the treatment.
• Check your child's head every two to three weeks.

SCABIES

Scabies is an irritating, itchy rash caused by a tiny mite. The burrowing and egg-laying of these mites produce a rash that nearly always affects the hands and fingers, particularly the clefts between the fingers. It may also affect the ankles, feet, toes, elbows and the area around the genitals. When the eggs hatch, they are easily passed to another person by direct contact. They can also be picked up from bedding or linen that is infested with the mites.

IS IT SERIOUS?

Scabies is not serious, but it is contagious and could run through a family or a school class if not treated promptly.

POSSIBLE SYMPTOMS

- Intense itchiness.
- Fine, short lines that end in a black spot the size of a pinhead, most often found between the fingers.
- Scabs on the itchy areas.

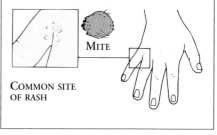

COMMON SITE OF RASH

MITE

WHAT SHOULD I DO FIRST?

1 If your child is scratching a lot, look for the fine lines of the mites' burrows.

2 If you suspect scabies, keep your child away from school until you have administered the treatment.

3 Try to discourage your child from scratching. This may hinder the doctor's diagnosis and cause sores to form that could become infected.

SHOULD I CONSULT THE DOCTOR?

Consult your doctor as soon as possible if you suspect scabies or if your child is scratching a lot.

WHAT MIGHT THE DOCTOR DO?

- Your doctor will prescribe a lotion in sufficient quantity for the whole family to be treated.
- Your doctor may prescribe an ointment to help the itchiness.

WHAT CAN I DO TO HELP?

- After thorough washing, you should paint the whole body below the neck with the lotion and leave to dry. Do not wash it off for 24 hours. To ensure disinfestation, repeat the procedure for a further 24 hours in a day or two.
- Carry out the treatment for other members of the family simultaneously.
- Launder or air all bedding and clothing to eradicate the mite. The mite does not live for longer than five or six days after it is removed from human skin.

SEE ALSO:
Itching, *page 35*

INGROWING TOENAIL

When a toenail fails to grow straight out from the nailbed, but instead curves over into the sides of the toe, it is referred to as an ingrowing toenail. This occurs most often to the nail of the big toe, and causes pain and discomfort. An ingrowing toenail is more likely to occur if the toe is broad and plump, if the toenail is cut down at the sides instead of straight across, if it is small, or if tight shoes and socks push the nail into the skin. If it is left untreated, the nail will penetrate the skin, possibly becoming infected, causing painful inflammation and a discharge of pus around the edges of the nail.

IS IT SERIOUS?

An ingrowing toenail can be painful but it is not serious.

WHAT SHOULD I DO FIRST?

1 Examine the skin around the nail to see if the nail has penetrated the skin.

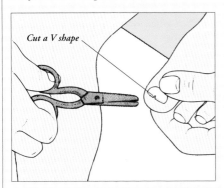

Cut a V shape

2 Cut a tiny V shape in the top edge of the nail to relieve pressure on the sides of the nail.

3 Apply an antiseptic cream to the sides of the nail to prevent infection.

4 If there is any sign of redness or pus, stop your child walking about and get him to lie down with his foot propped up. Apply a sterile dressing to the toe.

SHOULD I CONSULT THE DOCTOR?

Consult your doctor as soon as possible if the nail has penetrated the skin, if you notice any redness or pus around your child's toenail, or if ingrowing toenails are a recurrent problem.

WHAT MIGHT THE DOCTOR DO?

• Your doctor may prescribe antibiotic tablets to clear up the infection, and an antiseptic cream to apply to the affected area of the toe. Your doctor may also prescribe an astringent cream or lotion to toughen up the skin around the affected toenail.

• If the problem seems to be a recurrent one, your doctor may refer your child to an orthopaedic surgeon, so that he can examine him to see whether the ingrowing edge of the toenail should be removed. This is not a serious operation.

WHAT CAN I DO TO HELP?

INCORRECT   CORRECT

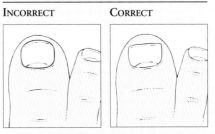

• Cut your child's toenails straight across and not too short. Cut them regularly.
• Make sure his shoes and socks are not too tight; allow him enough space to wriggle his toes.
• If his toenail becomes infected, don't put socks on him; cut the toe out of an old shoe or let him wear sandals while the infection is clearing up.

Verruca

A verruca is a wart on the sole of the foot that has been pushed up into the foot by the pressure of walking. It is highly infectious and is spread by direct contact with surfaces where people with infected feet have been going barefoot, such as communal swimming pools, showers and gymnasiums. It takes about two years for the body to build up resistance to the wart virus (after which the warts usually disappear naturally), but because a verruca can be spread easily and because it can be painful, treatment is always advisable.

IS IT SERIOUS?

A verruca is never serious but it can cause pain and discomfort, depending on where it appears on the sole of the foot.

POSSIBLE SYMPTOMS

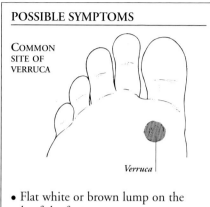

COMMON SITE OF VERRUCA

Verruca

- Flat white or brown lump on the sole of the foot.
- Pain when walking or standing on the foot.

WHAT SHOULD I DO FIRST?

1 Wash your child's feet and leave them to soak in warm water to soften the skin.

2 With a clean scalpel (available from the chemist) pare away thin layers of the softened verruca very gently. It is always wiser to take off too little rather than draw blood.

3 Apply a proprietary brand of wart treatment, obtainable from a chemist. Don't apply the wart treatment to healthy skin. To avoid this, use a corn plaster or a piece of ordinary plaster, with a hole the size of the verruca cut out of it, to protect the surrounding areas. After putting on the lotion, cover the verruca with a sterile dressing and plaster.

4 Repeat the procedure every day until the verruca has disappeared.

SHOULD I CONSULT THE DOCTOR?

Consult your doctor as soon as possible if the verruca is painful or if the verrucas are increasing in number, or if self-help treatment fails.

WHAT MIGHT THE DOCTOR DO?

Your doctor may refer you to a special wart clinic under the supervision of a dermatologist. The verruca will be removed either by treatment with a freezing agent such as liquid nitrogen, or by being burned off or scraped out under a local anaesthetic.

WHAT CAN I DO TO HELP?

- Cover the verruca completely with a secure plaster whenever your child goes barefoot; this should prevent the virus from spreading.
- Discourage your child from scratching the verruca. He could infect himself elsewhere.

CHAPTER 4

EYES, EARS, NOSE, THROAT & MOUTH

Young children are particularly susceptible to
infections of the eyes, ears, nose, throat and mouth,
because they have not yet built up immunity.
The entries in this chapter cover both childhood
ailments such as tonsillitis, as well as common
household accidents, like foreign bodies in the eye,
nose or ears. The emphasis is on sensible self-help
and practical advice about when you need help, so that
you can protect your child and help him recover.

DIAGNOSIS GUIDE

Young children are vulnerable to infections of the eyes, ears, nose and throat, and these organs are closely connected. To use this section, look for the symptom most similar to the one your child is suffering from then turn to the relevant entry. See also p. 13 for a list of emergency symptoms.

EARS

• **PAIN IN AND AROUND THE EAR**
possibly **Toothache**, see p. 80 or **Earache**, see p. 70 or **Otitis Externa**, see p. 71

• **IMPAIRED HEARING**
with fullness in the ear *possibly* **Glue ear**, see p. 69 or **Foreign body in Ear**, see p. 72

• **PAIN INSIDE THE EAR CANAL**
made worse when the earlobe is pulled *possibly* **Otitis externa**, see p. 71

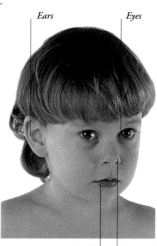

Ears   *Eyes*

Mouth | *Nose*

EYES

• **SORE, WATERY EYE**
possibly **Conjunctivitis**, see p. 77 or **Foreign body in Eye**, see p. 78. If accompanied by sneezing *possibly* **Hayfever**, see p. 89

• **PAIN UNDERNEATH THE EYES**
possibly **Sinusitis**, see p. 65

• **SWOLLEN, RED AREA**
on the eyelid, *possibly* **Stye**, see p. 75

• **PUS OOZING FROM THE INNER CORNER**
of the eye *possibly* **Sticky eye**, see p. 76

NOSE

• **BLEEDING NOSE**
possibly **Nosebleed**, see p. 74 or **Foreign body in nose**, see p. 73

MOUTH

• **RED OR WHITE SORE, ULCERATED AREA**
inside the mouth *possibly* **Mouth ulcer**, see p. 81

• **YELLOW OR WHITE FROTHY PATCHES**
in the mouth *possibly* oral **Thrush**, see p. 121

• **DESIRE TO BITE ON ANY HARD OBJECT**
accompanied by irritability and a swollen area on the gum in a young baby *possibly* **Teething**, see p. 79

• **RED, INFLAMED LUMP**
on the gum possibly with swollen glands *possibly* **Gum boil**, see p. 82, or in a young baby, **Teething**, see p. 79

COLD AND ALLERGY SYMPTOMS

SWOLLEN NECK GLANDS
accompanied by a fever *possibly* **Sore throat**, see p. 66, **Tonsillitis**, see p. 67 or **Laryngitis**, see p. 68
HOARSE COUGH OR LOSS OF VOICE
possibly **Croup**, see p. 88 or **Laryngitis**, see p. 68
DIARRHOEA, VOMITING OR NAUSEA
accompanied by shivering, fever and a cough *possibly* **Influenza**, see p, 87

SNEEZING, WITH A RUNNY NOSE
and itchy eyes *possibly* **Hayfever**, see p. 89
A RUNNY NOSE
often with a sore throat and fever *possibly* **Common cold**, see p. 63 or **Influenza**, see p. 87
RUNNY NOSE WITH A CLEAR DISCHARGE
and coughing, especially at night *possibly* **Catarrh**, see p. 64 or **Common cold**, see p. 63

COMMON COLD

The common cold is caused by a virus that enters the body through the nasal passages and throat and causes inflammation of the mucous membranes lining these passages. The body's defences take around ten days to fight off the virus.

IS IT SERIOUS?

A common cold is not serious. However, because it lowers the body's resistance, complications such as **bronchitis** can sometimes arise. A cold should be regarded more seriously in a baby because minor symptoms, such as a blocked nose, can cause feeding problems.

POSSIBLE SYMPTOMS

- Sneezing.
- Runny or blocked nose.
- Raised temperature.
- Coughing.
- Sore throat.
- Aching muscles.
- Irritability.
- Catarrh.

WHAT SHOULD I DO FIRST?

1 Take your child's temperature. If it is high, 38°C (100.4°F) or more, and it does not subside within four to five hours, put him to bed and bring his temperature down (see p. 15).

*2 Check your child's nasal discharge. Yellow discharge can indicate a secondary infection, while clear mucus could signify **hayfever**.*

3 Don't give any patent medicines without your doctor's advice.

SHOULD I CONSULT THE DOCTOR?

Consult your doctor immediately if you think your child has developed a secondary infection. If your baby is having trouble sleeping or feeding, consult your doctor or health visitor.

WHAT MIGHT THE DOCTOR DO?

- Your doctor will treat a secondary infection to the cold.
- Your doctor may prescribe nose drops to make feeding easier. Use as directed, as over-use can damage the nose lining.

- Your doctor may prescribe a cough suppressant or expectorant to ease a bad cough.

WHAT CAN I DO TO HELP?

- Ease your baby's breathing by placing a pillow under the mattress to raise his head.
- Give your child plenty to drink and teach him to blow his nose by blowing one nostril at a time.
- If possible, create a humid atmosphere in your child's bedroom.
- Smear Vaseline on to your child's nose and upper lip if they are sore.
- Capsules of camphor sprinkled on to clothing or bedding will ease your child's breathing during the night.
- A hot bedtime drink of fresh lemon juice and water will soothe your child's sore throat and clear his nasal passages.

SEE ALSO:
Bronchitis, *page 86*
Catarrh, *page 64*
Croup, *page 88*
Hayfever, *page 89*
Sore throat, *page 66*

CATARRH

Catarrh is an excess of mucus in the nose and throat. It may be the result of a **common cold** or occur with the onset of an infectious disease such as **measles**, or it may be a symptom of **influenza**. One of the most dramatic forms of acute catarrh occurs in **hayfever**, when the allergic reaction of a runny nose is accompanied by itchy, tearful eyes and sneezing.

Chronic catarrh may be caused by **sinusitis**. The mucus from the infected sinuses runs down the back of the throat, causing the child to cough, particularly when lying down. Breathing becomes difficult and, if a great deal of mucus is swallowed, this unpleasant sensation could lead to vomiting. Occasionally the symptoms of catarrh may also indicate a middle ear infection, enlarged adenoids or nasal polyps.

POSSIBLE SYMPTOMS

- Nasal congestion.
- Runny nose with a clear discharge.
- Coughing, especially at night.
- Difficulty in feeding in small babies.
- Vomiting if the mucus is swallowed.

IS IT SERIOUS?

Catarrh that accompanies a minor illness is not serious. However, chronic catarrh will require treatment.

WHAT SHOULD I DO FIRST?

1 Encourage your child to blow his nose frequently. The catarrh will probably not need any more treatment than this.

2 If your child is having difficulty breathing, apply a menthol rub to his chest or drops to his pillow at night. Or encourage him if he is old enough (over about ten), to inhale the fumes from menthol capsules dissolved in hot water.

3 If your child is coughing at night, prop him up with pillows, or raise the foot of the cot – a telephone directory under it would be about the right elevation – so that the mucus doesn't drip down his throat.

4 Never use nose drops without your doctor's advice.

SHOULD I CONSULT THE DOCTOR?

Consult your doctor as soon as possible if the catarrh is making feeding difficult for your baby. Consult him as soon as possible if you think the catarrh may be an allergic reaction, such as hayfever, or if it persists for no apparent reason.

WHAT MIGHT THE DOCTOR DO?

- For a baby, your doctor may prescribe nose drops to relieve the congestion.
- If he thinks it is caused by an allergy, he will probably test for possible causes.
- If the catarrh is caused by chronic sinusitis or middle ear infection, antibiotics will be prescribed. If it is caused by enlarged adenoids or nasal polyps, surgical removal may be recommended.

WHAT CAN I DO TO HELP?

Teach your child to blow his nose by clearing out one nostril at a time.

SEE ALSO:
Common cold, *page 63*
Hayfever, *page 89*
Influenza, *page 87*
Measles, *page 28*
Sinusitis, *page 65*

SINUSITIS

Sinusitis is a bacterial infection of the cheek and forehead sinuses. These air-filled spaces, grouped around the eyes and nose, make the skull bones light, and give the voice resonance. Infections of the sinuses are rare in babies because their sinuses are not fully developed, but in older children some degree of sinusitis often accompanies a **common cold, cough** or **sore throat.**

A yellow-green discharge of pus from the nose is often the sign that your child has sinusitis.

IS IT SERIOUS?

Sinusitis is not a serious ailment, although it can become chronic if it is not treated efficiently when it first appears.

POSSIBLE SYMPTOMS

- Yellow-green discharge of pus from the nose where previously there was a clear, runny discharge.
- Pain over the cheeks.
- Pain on moving the head.
- Slight fever.
- Blocked nose.

AFFECTED AREAS

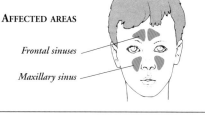

Frontal sinuses

Maxillary sinus

WHAT SHOULD I DO FIRST?

1 If your child has a cold, cough or a sore throat, watch out for a change in the colour of his nasal discharge.

*2 Check to see if there is a **foreign body** lodged in your child's nose. The discharge will then be foul-smelling and stained with blood. Seek medical help immediately if you cannot easily remove the foreign body.*

3 If there is no foreign object, relieve his blocked nose by encouraging him if he is old enough (over about ten) to inhale the fumes of menthol capsules dissolved in boiling water.

SHOULD I CONSULT THE DOCTOR?

Consult your doctor as soon as possible if the yellow-green nasal discharge continues for more than two days.

WHAT MIGHT THE DOCTOR DO?

- Your doctor will prescribe antibiotics to eradicate the infection. He may also prescribe special nose drops for your child to take whenever he has a cold, so that the sinuses keep draining, thus preventing a recurrence of sinusitis.
- If the infection persists, he will prescribe a course of antibiotics to prevent it from becoming chronic.
- If sinusitis is recurrent, your doctor will refer your child to an ear, nose and throat specialist to see whether surgical draining of the sinuses is necessary.

WHAT CAN I DO TO HELP?

- If your child complains of a headache or fever, give him liquid paracetamol.
- Continue giving your child menthol inhalations to relieve the symptoms.
- Don't overheat your child's bedroom. Keep the air cool and humid; a dry atmosphere makes the symptoms worse.

SEE ALSO:
Common cold, *page 63*
Cough, *page 85*
Nose, foreign body in, *page 73*
Sore throat, *page 66*

SORE THROAT

A sore throat is usually a symptom of an infection of the respiratory tract. While a baby or young child may not be able to tell you about the raw feeling in his throat, you will notice that he has difficulty swallowing. Sore throats can occur because of inflammation of the tonsils (**tonsillitis**), caused by the *streptococcus* bacterium, or more usually by a virus, such as the **common cold** or **influenza**. If there is inflammation elsewhere, as there is in the larynx when your child has **laryngitis**, this can also give a raw feeling in the throat. If the glands in the neck are swollen, with **mumps**, for example, this may be felt by your child as pain in the throat.

IS IT SERIOUS?

Most sore throats are not serious. However, if your child is allergic to the *streptococcus* bacterium and he has a streptococcal infection in the throat, this could have effects elsewhere in his body. Occasional more serious complications that can occur include illnesses such as nephritis and rheumatic fever.

WHAT SHOULD I DO FIRST?

1 If your child complains of a sore throat, or if he is having difficulty swallowing and is off his food, carefully examine his throat in a good light, with his head held back and the tongue depressed gently with the handle of a clean spoon. Ask him to say a long "aaah". This will open up the throat wide enough so that you will be able to check to see if there is any inflammation or if the tonsils are enlarged.

2 Gently run your fingers down either side of your child's neck and under his chin to check if he has any swelling in the glands – the glands should feel like large peas under the skin.

*3 Take your child's temperature to see if he has a **fever**.*

4 As the sore throat is most likely to be caused by some sort of infection, keep your child away from school or nursery school until you have seen your doctor and obtained confirmation that it is not contagious.

SHOULD I CONSULT THE DOCTOR?

Consult your doctor as soon as possible. Streptococcal infection of the throat should be treated promptly to avoid complications.

WHAT MIGHT THE DOCTOR DO?

Your doctor will examine your child to determine the cause of the sore throat. If it is a *streptococcus* bacterium, he will prescribe antibiotics.

WHAT CAN I DO TO HELP?

• Soothe your child's sore throat with cold drinks or hot lemon drinks.
• Give your child plenty of liquids. If he isn't eating because it hurts to swallow, liquidize foods where possible.

SEE ALSO:
Common cold, *page 63*
Fever, *page 25*
Influenza, *page 87*
Laryngitis, *page 68*
Mumps, *page 29*
Tonsillitis, *page 67*

TONSILLITIS

Positioned at the back of the throat, the tonsils are the body's first line of defence. They trap and kill bacteria, preventing them from entering the respiratory tract. In the process, they can become infected, causing tonsillitis. The adenoids, at the back of the nose, are usually affected as well.

Babies under the age of about one rarely suffer from tonsillitis; it occurs mainly among school-age children, when the relatively large tonsils and adenoids are exposed to infectious microbes. As resistance to infectious microbes increases, attacks should lessen. Most children do not get tonsillitis after the age of ten.

IS IT SERIOUS?

Tonsillitis is not serious unless repeatedly accompanied by infection of the middle ear.

POSSIBLE SYMPTOMS

- Sore throat, possibly bad enough to cause difficulty in swallowing.
- Red and enlarged tonsils, possibly covered in yellow spots.
- A temperature of over 38°C (100.4°F).
- Swollen glands in the neck.
- Mouth-breathing, snoring and a nasal voice.
- Unpleasant breath.

AREA AFFECTED

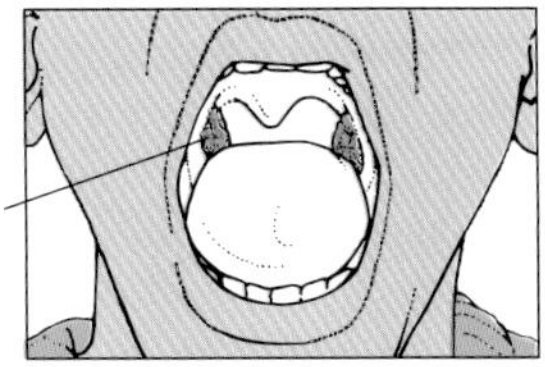

WHAT SHOULD I DO FIRST?

1 *If your child has a sore throat or difficulty eating, check his throat. Ask him to say a long "aaah". You should be able to see if his tonsils are red, enlarged or covered with spots.*

2 *Take your child's temperature to see if he has a* ***fever****, and check to see if his glands are swollen – they will feel like large peas under the skin.*

3 *Ask him if he has earache. In a young child, note whether he pulls or rubs his ears. Check to see if there is any discharge.*

SHOULD I CONSULT THE DOCTOR?

Consult your doctor as soon as possible if you suspect tonsillitis.

WHAT MIGHT THE DOCTOR DO?

- Your doctor may take a throat swab to identify the infection. He may prescribe antibiotics for bacterial tonsillitis.
- He will examine your child's ears to check for any infection. If there are any signs he will prescribe antibiotics.
- If your child suffers from frequent tonsillitis attacks, or if enlarged adenoids cause recurrent middle-ear infections, you may be referred to a specialist.

WHAT CAN I DO TO HELP?

- Treat your child as you would for fever.
- Keep your child's fluid intake up by offering regular drinks.
- Never give your child a gargle for a sore throat. It can spread infection from the throat to the middle ear.
- Offer him foods that slip down easily, but don't force him to eat.

SEE ALSO:
Earache, *page 70*
Fever, *page 25*
Sore throat, *page 66*

LARYNGITIS

Laryngitis is an inflammation of the larynx, or voice box. Many minor viruses, and occasionally bacteria, can enter the body through the throat and quickly infect the larynx. The most obvious symptoms of laryngitis are hoarseness and a dry **cough**, and sometimes **fever**.

IS IT SERIOUS?

Laryngitis is rarely serious and lasts less than seven days, even if it is part of a more serious infection, such as **tonsillitis** or **bronchitis**. However, in young children a swollen larynx can obstruct the passage of air, causing breathing difficulties and **croup**, which is a serious complication. If laryngitis develops into croup, you should seek urgent medical treatment.

POSSIBLE SYMPTOMS

- Hoarseness or loss of voice.
- Dry cough.
- Slight fever.
- Sore throat.
- Croup, a type of barking cough.

CROSS-SECTION OF THE THROAT

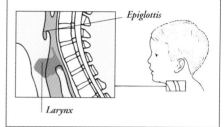

Epiglottis

Larynx

WHAT SHOULD I DO FIRST?

1 *If the hoarseness is not accompanied by any other symptoms of respiratory tract infection, such as bronchitis, keep a check on your child's temperature. If it rises above 38°C (100.4°F), there may be another infection present.*

2 *Listen closely for the barking cough of croup.*

3 *Keep the air in your child's room moist if possible. Open a window to allow air to circulate. This is usually an effective atmosphere for suppressing a dry cough.*

SHOULD I CONSULT THE DOCTOR?

Consult your doctor immediately if you think your child has croup. Consult your doctor as soon as possible if your child has a fever or you think he has contracted another infection.

WHAT MIGHT THE DOCTOR DO?

If there is a bacterial infection such as bronchitis or tonsillitis, your doctor will prescribe antibiotics.

WHAT CAN I DO TO HELP?

- Discourage your child from talking out loud. You could make a game of it and have the whole family talking in whispers.
- Give your child plenty of warm drinks to soothe his throat. Try hot lemon and honey or heat any fruit juice drink by diluting it with hot water.

SEE ALSO:
Bronchitis, *page 86*
Cough, *page 85*
Croup, *page 88*
Fever, *page 25*
Tonsillitis, *page 67*

GLUE EAR

Glue ear is a condition that results when the Eustachian tube and middle ear are filled with fluid as a result of infection. The Eustachian tube, which runs from the throat to the ear, produces large quantities of fluid as a response to chronic infections such as **sinusitis**, **tonsillitis**, or, most commonly, infection of the middle ear. If the tube in either ear is blocked by inflammmation, the fluid cannot drain and becomes glue-like, impeding the efficient vibration of sound, causing loss of hearing.

IS IT SERIOUS?

Glue ear should be treated seriously because it can lead to permanent loss of hearing in the affected ear, and can cause problems with speech development and learning.

POSSIBLE SYMPTOMS

- A feeling of fullness in the ear.
- Partial loss of hearing or deafness in one or both ears.

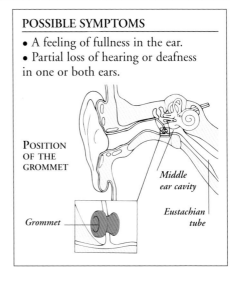

POSITION OF THE GROMMET

Middle ear cavity

Eustachian tube

Grommet

WHAT SHOULD I DO FIRST?

If your child seems inattentive and has recently had a cold, do a hearing test. Call quietly when his head is averted and see if there is a response. Even if he can hear you, the hearing may be impaired in such a way that he cannot tell where you are calling from.

SHOULD I CONSULT THE DOCTOR?

Consult your doctor as soon as possible.

WHAT MIGHT THE DOCTOR DO?

- Your doctor will examine your child's ears with a special instrument called an otoscope.
- In mild cases, your doctor will prescribe antibiotics to clear up the infection, and he may also prescribe vasoconstrictor drugs, which promote drainage by reducing swelling in the Eustachian tubes.
- In severe and recurrent cases, your child will probably be referred to an ear, nose and throat specialist for a hearing

test. He may be admitted to hospital to have the fluid drained off under a general anaesthetic and grommets may be inserted. These are tiny plastic tubes that allow mucus to drain away. They either fall out after several months when the ears are healthy again, or can be removed by the specialist. If glue ear is a result of repeated infections or enlarged adenoids, the underlying problem will also be treated to prevent recurrences.

WHAT CAN I DO TO HELP?

- If your child has had grommets inserted, he must always wear a bathing cap when swimming and should not dive. Some doctors advise against swimming.
- Try to keep the ear as dry as possible.

SEE ALSO:
Common cold, *page 63*
Sinusitis, *page 65*
Tonsillitis, *page 67*

EARACHE

There are a number of causes of earache. The most common is *otitis media* an infection of the middle ear. This is especially true in children under six, because the tube that runs from the throat to the ear – the Eustachian tube – is relatively short, and infections of the nose and throat can be easily spread to the middle ear cavity. A child may complain of earache if he is suffering from **toothache**, **tonsillitis** or **mumps**; when the glands in his neck are swollen; or if he has been out in a cold wind without protective headgear. Earache with an intense pain will result from an infection of the outer ear (**otitis externa**) if, for example, a **foreign body** has been poked into the ear or if a **boil** has developed.

POSSIBLE SYMPTOMS

- Pain in the area around the ear.
- A temperature of over 38°C (100.4°F).
- Discharge of pus from the ear.
- Deafness.
- Inflammation of the tonsils.
- Pain when the ear is touched.
- Swollen glands.
- Rubbing and pulling of the ear in a young child.

IS IT SERIOUS?

Earache with loss of hearing is serious. If the condition is not treated, it could cause permanent damage to the middle ear.

WHAT SHOULD I DO FIRST?

1 Take your child's temperature to see if he has a fever.

2 Check whether there is any discharge from the ear and whether your child's hearing is diminished. To do this, call his name quietly when his head is averted. See if he turns around.

3 Examine the back of your child's throat to see if the tonsils are abnormally enlarged or red.

4 Check to see if there is any inflammation in the outer ear cavity. Do not put even a cotton-wool swab into the ear or use eardrops unless your doctor advises it.

SHOULD I CONSULT THE DOCTOR?

Consult your doctor as soon as possible if your child complains of earache; most earache is caused by infection. Consult him immediately if your child is in pain and has a high fever, especially if you notice any discharge from the ear.

Consult him immediately if your child is too young to tell you he's in pain but is crying, and pulling or rubbing an ear.

WHAT MIGHT THE DOCTOR DO?

Your doctor will examine your child to determine the cause of the earache. If it is caused by a bacterial infection, he will probably prescribe antibiotics.

WHAT SHOULD I DO TO HELP?

- Place a hot-water bottle, covered by a towel, next to your child's ear to relieve pain, unless the source of the earache is a boil, or give him paracetamol.
- Prevent water from entering the ear during bathing.

SEE ALSO:
Boil, *page 47*
Ear, foreign body in, *page 72*
Mumps, *page 29*
Otitis externa, *page 71*
Tonsillitis, *page 67*
Toothache, *page 80*

OTITIS EXTERNA

Otitis externa is an infection of the external ear canal – the passage that leads from the ear flap (pinna) to the eardrum. The infection may be caused by a **foreign body** in the ear, by a **boil** in the canal, or as the result of damage to the skin from over-vigorous cleaning or scratching. The infection is more common in children who swim a great deal.

POSSIBLE SYMPTOMS

- Earache.
- Redness and tenderness of the ear flap and external ear canal.
- Pus-filled boil in the canal.
- Discharge from the ear.
- Itchy, dry, scaly ear.

IS IT SERIOUS?

As the external ear canal does not contain the ear's delicate hearing mechanisms, the infection itself is relatively minor. However, it will always be treated because in rare cases the infection could spread to the skull bones, and possibly the brain. Any discharge from the ear should be treated seriously as this could be a symptom of a serious middle ear infection.

WHAT SHOULD I DO FIRST?

1 Look into the external ear canal to check for any signs of infection or foreign objects. Remove the objects if you can do so easily. Do not push or poke anything into your child's ear, and discourage him from touching or scratching it if it's sore.

2 Ask your child to open his mouth wide to see if this causes pain.

3 Pull back gently on the ear flap to see if this causes pain. Clean away any discharge with warm water and soap.

4 Give your child paracetamol to relieve pain, and place a cotton-wool pad over the ear to absorb any discharge.

SHOULD I CONSULT THE DOCTOR?

Consult your doctor as soon as possible if you notice any discharge from your child's ear or if you suspect infection.

WHAT MIGHT THE DOCTOR DO?

- Your doctor will examine your child's ear with a special instrument called an otoscope, and may then clean out the ear with a probe. He will probably prescribe antibiotic ear drops or tablets to clear up the infection.
- If there is a foreign body in your child's ear, your doctor will remove it or refer him to hospital for its removal.
- If the pain is the result of a boil, he may lance it and drain the pus away.

WHAT CAN I DO TO HELP?

- If your child is in pain, give him paracetamol on the advice of your doctor.
- Prevent water from entering the ear until the infection has cleared. Don't let your child go swimming.
- Don't interfere with your child's external ear canal; never poke cotton-wool swabs into it to clear wax, for example. They will only push it further into the canal or damage the lining.
- Never use patent eardrops unless your doctor advises them.

SEE ALSO:
Boil, *page 47*
Earache, *page 70*
Ear, foreign body in, *page 72*

EAR, FOREIGN BODY IN

The most common foreign bodies to become stuck in a child's ear are small objects, like beads, pushed in by the child or by a playmate. Very rarely, a small insect may fly into the ear and be trapped there.

IS IT SERIOUS?

Any foreign body in the ear that cannot be removed easily should be regarded as serious because it may cause an infection of the external ear canal, **otitis externa**, or damage the eardrum.

POSSIBLE SYMPTOMS

- Pain and tenderness in the ear.
- A visible embedded object.

WHAT SHOULD I DO?

1 If the object is small and soft, try to remove it with tweezers. If you can't grasp it without poking in the ear, leave it and consult your doctor immediately.

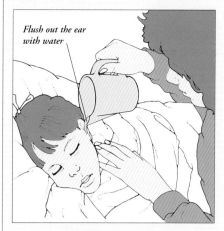

Flush out the ear with water

2 If the foreign body is an insect, lay your child on his side with the affected ear uppermost and pour warm water into the ear. The insect should float out.

SHOULD I CONSULT THE DOCTOR?

Consult your doctor immediately if the object cannot be removed, or if your child complains of pain and tenderness in the ear.

WHAT MIGHT THE DOCTOR DO?

After examining your child's external ear canal, your doctor will remove the object and will treat any damage to the skin, or any infection that may have been caused by the foreign body.

WHAT CAN I DO TO HELP?

Don't let a child under three play with small objects which he could poke into his ear – or into his nose or mouth.

SEE ALSO:
Otitis externa, *page 71*

NOSE, FOREIGN BODY IN

If there is a foreign body of any sort in your child's nose, it is most likely to have been pushed in there by your child or a playmate. The problem may not even be noticed by you or your child at first, but after two or three days there will probably be a **nosebleed**, or perhaps even a blood-stained, foul-smelling discharge from the affected nostril.

IS IT SERIOUS?

If the foreign body cannot be easily removed from your child's nose, on no account attempt to remove it yourself – you might push it further in. Instead, you should consult your doctor immediately or take your child to your nearest hospital casualty department.

POSSIBLE SYMPTOMS

- Nosebleeds.
- Smelly, blood-stained discharge from the nostril.
- Red, swollen, tender area over the nose.
- Peculiar odour on your child's breath, sometimes said to smell like ripe cheese.

If the foreign body can be easily removed , it is not serious and should have no after-effects. It is more serious if your child inhales the object into his lungs, as this may partially block his air passages and result in breathing difficulties, **croup** or **choking**.

WHAT SHOULD I DO FIRST?

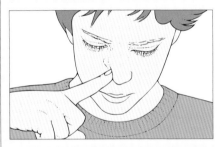

1 If your child is old enough to under-stand, ask him to hold a finger against the good nostril and blow the affected one to dislodge the foreign body. Don't ask a young child to do this – he might sniff the object back into his air passages.

2 Or, lay your child on his back and shine a light on his face. If you can see the object near the entrance to the nose, and if it is soft, remove it with tweezers. If it moves further up the nostril, leave it alone. If your child has breathing problems, treat this as an emergency.

SHOULD I CONSULT THE DOCTOR?

Consult your doctor immediately or take your child to the nearest hospital casualty department if you cannot easily remove a foreign body from his nose.

WHAT MIGHT THE DOCTOR DO?

Your doctor will remove the foreign body with a pair of forceps. If your child is very young, or refuses to stay still, he may have to be taken to hospital to have it removed under general anaesthetic.

WHAT CAN I DO TO HELP?

Try not to allow a child under the age of three to play with toys or objects small enough to swallow or put up his nose.

SEE ALSO:
Choking, *page 92*
Croup, *page 88*
Nosebleed, *page 74*

NOSEBLEED

A nosebleed occurs when a small area of blood vessels on the inner surface of the nose ruptures. This can be caused by hard blowing or even sneezing when your child has a **common cold** or **hayfever**, for instance, by a knock on the nose, by picking the nose, or by a **foreign body** in the nose; in this last case, the blood will be accompanied by a blood-stained, foul-smelling discharge. The blood loss from a nosebleed can look very dramatic, but is usually very little.

IS IT SERIOUS?

A nosebleed is rarely serious. But if your child has frequent nosebleeds that don't stop easily, or if his nose bleeds after a blow to the head, medical help should be sought.

WHAT SHOULD I DO FIRST?

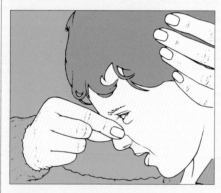

1 Don't try to staunch the blood by pushing anything into the nostrils. Sit your child down with his head forward over a basin or sink.

2 Apply firm pressure to both nostrils, gripping his nose between your thumb and forefinger just where the bone ends. Squeeze until the bleeding stops. Don't let him put his head back during a nosebleed. This allows blood to drip down the back of the nose into the stomach and can cause irritation and vomiting.

SHOULD I CONSULT THE DOCTOR?

Consult your doctor immediately if the nosebleed fails to stop after 30 minutes and your child is dizzy. Consult him urgently if there is a foreign body in your child's nose, or if the bleeds are frequent.

WHAT MIGHT THE DOCTOR DO?

• If your child has suffered a blow to the head, your doctor will probably arrange for an X-ray to discount the possibility of a fractured skull.
• If the nosebleed has failed to stop, your doctor will pack your child's nose with gauze to stem the blood flow. This will be done under a local anaesthetic. The gauze can be removed after a couple of hours.
• If your child has a foreign object stuck in his nose, your doctor will remove it, under local anaesthetic if necessary.
• If the nosebleeds are frequent, your doctor may refer you to an ear, nose and throat specialist for assessment. If the recurrent nosebleeds are caused by a fragile blood vessel, the specialist may cauterize it. This involves burning off the end of the vessel, and is done under a general anaesthetic.

WHAT CAN I DO TO HELP?

Don't let your child blow his nose for at least three hours after a nosebleed; the bleeding might start again.

SEE ALSO
Common cold, *page 63*
Hayfever, *page 89*
Nose, foreign body in, *page 73*

STYE

A stye is a pus-filled swelling on the margin of the eyelid. It is caused by an infection of one of the hair follicles from which the eyelashes grow, and it nearly always appears on the lower eyelid. It usually comes to a head and bursts within four or five days. Styes are encouraged by rubbing and pulling at the eyelashes and may also be associated with a general inflammation of the eyelids known as blepharitis. Styes are not highly infectious, but they can be spread from one eye to the other.

IS IT SERIOUS?

A stye is usually harmless and can be treated at home.

POSSIBLE SYMPTOMS

• Swollen, sore red area on the eyelid, which enlarges to become pus-filled.
• Rubbing and pulling at eyelashes, accompanied by irritation of the eye.

COMMON SITE

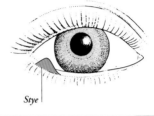

Stye

WHAT SHOULD I DO FIRST?

1 If the spot on the eyelid is merely red and sore, leave it alone and discourage your child from rubbing it. If it is painful and unsightly, keep it still with gauze held loosely in place with a bandage.

2 If the stye is pus-filled and painful, apply a ball of cotton wool squeezed out in hot water for a few minutes every two or three hours. This will soothe the pain and bring the stye to a head.

3 Once the stye has come to a head, try to release the pus and ease the pain by gently pulling out the lash at the centre of the stye with a pair of tweezers. If it won't come out, leave it, and continue with the warm compresses. As soon as the lash comes out, the pus will drain away and the stye will get better quickly. Bathe the pus away with warm water and cotton wool.

4 Note whether the eyelids are red rimmed, with dandruff-like flakes clinging to the eyelashes. This could be blepharitis.

SHOULD I CONSULT THE DOCTOR?

Consult your doctor as soon as possible if the home treatment does not improve the stye within four or five days, or if the eyelid becomes generally swollen, or if the stye is accompanied by blepharitis.

WHAT MIGHT THE DOCTOR DO?

If there is an infection of the eyelid or the eye itself, your doctor will prescribe an antibiotic ointment or eye drops. If the stye is accompanied by blepharitis, your doctor may prescribe an ointment to clear it up.

WHAT CAN I DO TO HELP?

• Keep your child's facecloth and towel separate from those of the rest of the family to avoid spreading any infection.
• Wash your hands before and after treating the stye and discourage your child from touching the area.

STICKY EYE

Sticky eye is a mild infection that is quite common during the first week of a baby's life. It is nearly always due to a foreign substance getting into the eye during delivery, possibly a drop of amniotic fluid or blood. Your baby's eye will ooze pus and when he wakes up, the eye will be gummed up.

IS IT SERIOUS?

Sticky eye is not a serious complaint. It poses no danger to your baby's eyes, but the ailment should nevertheless be treated promptly to prevent the more serious complaint of the eye membrane, **conjunctivitis**, from developing.

POSSIBLE SYMPTOMS

- Pus coming from the inner corner of one or both of the eyes.
- Eyelashes stuck together after sleep.

WHAT SHOULD I DO FIRST?

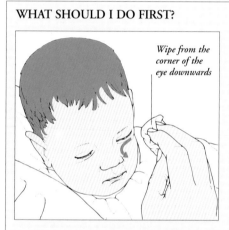

Wipe from the corner of the eye downwards

1 Wash both eyes with warm, boiled water, using a clean piece of cotton wool for each eye. Start on the outside corner of the eye and move downwards.

2 Put your baby down to sleep with the infected eye uppermost. The other eye may otherwise become infected from the sheet.

SHOULD I CONSULT THE DOCTOR?

Consult your doctor immediately if your baby's eyeball is red. This could be conjunctivitis. Consult your doctor as soon as possible if the sticky eye does not improve within 24 hours.

WHAT MIGHT THE DOCTOR DO?

If there is an infection, your doctor will prescribe eye drops or an eye ointment that can be applied to the eye three or four times a day.

WHAT CAN I DO TO HELP?

- Bathe your baby's eyes frequently, whenever you notice a discharge.
- Change his bed sheets regularly after every sleep (particularly his pillowcases) to avoid infecting the unaffected eye.

SEE ALSO:
Conjunctivitis, *page 77*

CONJUNCTIVITIS

Conjunctivitis is an inflammation of the *conjunctiva*, which is the membrane covering the eyeball and the inside of the eyelid. The inflammation may be caused by a viral or bacterial infection, or by injury from a **foreign body** or chemicals, or it may be the result of an allergic reaction. The eyes become red and weepy, and they can be painful, very itchy and irritated by bright light. The condition, which may affect one or both eyes, is contagious.

IS IT SERIOUS?

Although conjunctivitis is not serious, it should always be treated by a doctor.

POSSIBLE SYMPTOMS

- Weepy, red eyes that feel sore or itchy.
- Intolerance of bright light.
- Discharge of pus causing eyelashes to stick together after a night's sleep.

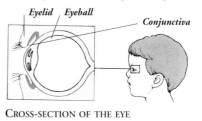

Eyelid   Eyeball   *Conjunctiva*

CROSS-SECTION OF THE EYE

WHAT SHOULD I DO FIRST?

1 Check to see if there is a foreign body in the eye; if possible remove it (see p. 78).

2 Before consulting your doctor, bathe each eye, whether both are affected or not, with a solution of 5ml (1 teaspoonful) salt dissolved in a glass of warm, previously boiled, water. Using a new cotton wool ball for each eye, soak it in the solution, then wipe from the inner corner of the eye outwards.

3 If only one eye is affected, you can use an eye pad to prevent rubbing and further friction between the conjunctiva *and other parts of the eye. Make sure that the eye pad itself does not aggravate the infection. Use a gauze pad held in place by a bandage.*

4 To prevent the spread of infection, encourage your child to keep his hands clean and not to rub his eyes.

SHOULD I CONSULT THE DOCTOR?

Consult your doctor as soon as possible if you suspect conjunctivitis.

WHAT MIGHT THE DOCTOR DO?

- If the condition is caused by an infection, your doctor will prescribe antibiotic eye drops or ointment to clear it. If the infection does not respond to treatment within a few days, your doctor may refer you to an eye specialist.
- If the irritation is caused by an allergy, such as **hayfever**, your doctor will prescribe anti-inflammatory eye drops and antihistamine medication.
- If there is a foreign body in your child's eye, your doctor will remove it.

WHAT CAN I DO TO HELP?

- Make your child understand that to prevent the infection from spreading, he should always keep his hands clean; he should also use a separate facecloth and towel.
- If your child suffers from hayfever, keep him away from freshly mown lawns during the worst hayfever months.

SEE ALSO:
Eye, foreign body in, *page 78*
Hayfever, *page 89*

Eye, Foreign Body In

If a foreign body such as a speck of dust or grit enters your child's eye, it will water and your child will not want to open it. If you can see something moving loosely over the white part, you can try to remove it. If, however, the foreign body is embedded in the eyeball or is on the coloured part of the eye (the iris), don't touch it.

POSSIBLE SYMPTOMS

- Watery eye.
- Reluctance to open the eye.
- Pain and irritation.
- A visible embedded object.

IS IT SERIOUS?

Small specks of dust or grit in the eye are not serious as they are washed out naturally by the tears, but if your child's eyeball is scratched, if an object has pierced it, or if there is any kind of cut on the eyeball or eyelid, this is serious and you should take him to your nearest hospital casualty department for treatment.

WHAT SHOULD I DO FIRST?

Look closely to see whether the foreign body is moving or embedded in the eye. Encourage your child to blink a few times – this may dislodge it, as may tears if he has been crying because of the pain and irritation.

If the foreign body is embedded in the eye

1 Do not attempt first aid. Keep your child's eye closed by putting a pad over the eyelid and taping it securely in place. Go straight to the nearest casualty department for treatment.

If the foreign body is not embedded in the eye

1 Ask your child to look upwards. Pull down the eyelid to see if the object is there. If it is, remove it with the corner of a clean handkerchief.

2 Expose the area beneath the top lid, by holding the eyelashes and pulling them back. Remove the object with the corner of a handkerchief. If your child won't co-operate, you will need someone to help you. Take him to the doctor if he resists.

3 If these methods don't work, try to flush the foreign body out by pouring a glass of water, to which you have added a pinch of salt, across the open eye.

SHOULD I CONSULT THE DOCTOR?

Go immediately to the nearest casualty department if the eyeball is scratched or if a foreign body has pierced the eye. Consult your doctor immediately if you cannot easily remove a floating foreign body from your child's eye. Consult your doctor as soon as possible if your child still complains of pain an hour or two after you have removed the object.

WHAT MIGHT THE DOCTOR DO?

- The hospital doctor will remove an embedded foreign body from your child's eye after putting drops of a local anaesthetic into the eye.
- If the eyeball is scratched, the doctor will prescribe antibiotic drops to guard against infection and may bandage the eye to keep it closed for about 24 hours.
- If you went to your doctor because your child's eye was still sore, your doctor will examine the eye and remove any foreign object that he finds.

TEETHING

Teething is the term used to describe the eruption of a baby's first teeth. Teething usually begins at about the age of six or seven months, with most of the first teeth breaking through before your baby is 18 months old. Your baby will produce more saliva than usual and will dribble; he will try to cram his fingers into his mouth and chew on his fingers or any other object that he can get hold of. He may be clingy and irritable, have difficulty sleeping, and he may cry and fret more than usual. Most of these symptoms occur just before the teeth erupt. It is important to realize that the symptoms of teething do not include bronchitis, nappy rash, vomiting, diarrhoea or loss of appetite. These are symptoms of an underlying illness, *not* teething.

IS IT SERIOUS?

Teething and the symptoms associated with teething are never serious.

POSSIBLE SYMPTOMS

• Increased saliva and dribbling.
• Desire to bite on any hard object.
• Irritability and increased clinginess.
• Sleeplessness.
• Swollen red area where the tooth is being cut.

ORDER OF APPEARANCE

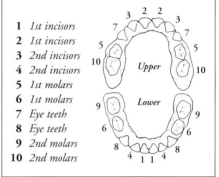

1 *1st incisors*
2 *1st incisors*
3 *2nd incisors*
4 *2nd incisors*
5 *1st molars*
6 *1st molars*
7 *Eye teeth*
8 *Eye teeth*
9 *2nd molars*
10 *2nd molars*

WHAT SHOULD I DO FIRST?

If you can't work out why your child is so irritable, feel his gums. If a tooth is coming through, you will feel a hard, sharp lump and the gum area will be swollen and red.

SHOULD I CONSULT THE DOCTOR?

You should not need to consult your doctor unless your child has other symptoms that cannot be attributed to teething.

WHAT MIGHT THE DOCTOR DO?

Your doctor will give you advice on how to cope with the symptoms of teething and may prescribe a mild analgesic to relieve the pain.

WHAT CAN I DO TO HELP?

• Nurse your baby often. A teething baby needs comfort and closeness. The arrival of teeth doesn't mean a necessary speeding-up of the weaning process. Babies with teeth can still be breastfed, with no discomfort to the mother.
• Distract your child with a chilled teething ring (never freeze it or your baby may get frostbite) or a piece of carrot – something with a firm texture. Never leave him with food in case he chokes.
• Try not to resort to giving your baby paracetamol. Over the course of the teething process, doses of such pain relievers could become too large. Only use pain relief on your doctor's advice.
• Rub the swollen gum with your finger. Try to avoid teething jellies that contain local anaesthetics as they have only a temporary effect and can sometimes cause allergy.
• If your child refuses food, encourage him to eat by giving him cold, smooth foods such as yoghurt, ice cream or jelly.

TOOTHACHE

Toothache is the pain that results when a tooth is decaying. The decaying process erodes the outer protective coatings of the tooth and bores through to the nerves in the soft centre, causing pain, particularly when anything cold, hot or sweet touches the tooth. Tooth decay and gum disease are caused by plaque, a thin film of saliva and food residue in which bacteria grow. The bacteria thrive in the presence of sugar in the mouth, which is one of the reasons why sugar in the diet is so harmful. Teeth can become resistant to the action of bacteria and sugar if they contain fluoride or if they are painted or coated with fluoride as they would be if regularly brushed with a fluoride-containing toothpaste. This is one of the main ways to prevent tooth decay, along with good oral hygiene and regular dental check-ups. It is important that children do not lose their first teeth through tooth decay, or a **gum boil**, a complication of tooth decay which the root of the tooth also decays. The permanent tooth may come through misaligned if a gap is left for too long while the new tooth is developing.

IS IT SERIOUS?

Toothache is not serious as long as it is treated immediately. If untreated, a gum boil may erupt, causing damage to the underlying permanent tooth, or loss of a second tooth.

WHAT SHOULD I DO FIRST?

*1 If your child complains of pain in the jaw, **earache**, or throbbing pains in the mouth, tap his teeth with a metal spoon to see if this identifies the source of the pain.*

2 Give him paracetamol to relieve the pain until you can visit the dentist. Or put a hot-water bottle covered in a towel against his cheek.

3 Do not apply oil of cloves or anaesthetic jellies as they can cause damage to the gum around the tooth.

SHOULD I CONSULT THE DOCTOR?

You don't need to consult a doctor, but you should consult your dentist immediately for an emergency appointment.

WHAT MIGHT THE DENTIST DO?

Your dentist will examine the tooth. It may only need to be drilled and filled, but if there is a gum boil he will drain the pus from the abscess. If he cannot save the tooth, it will be extracted, probably under a general anaesthetic, although this will depend on the age of your child.

WHAT CAN I DO TO HELP?

• Prevent tooth decay. Use fluoride toothpastes and fluoride tablets or drops in your child's drinks if your water is not already fluoridated.
• Restrict your child's sugar intake. Don't give him sweets, cakes and biscuits, and avoid canned foods and fizzy drinks.
• Brush your child's teeth yourself once a day or supervise the brushing.
• Once your child is four, take him for a dental check-up every six months to get him used to the dentist early.
• Encourage your child to drink lots of water after eating sweet foods, to wash most of the sugar off his teeth.
• Ask your dentist about fissure sealing.

SEE ALSO:
Earache, *page 70*
Gum boil, *page 82*

MOUTH ULCER

Children suffer from a variety of mouth ulcers, all of them painful, though most are relatively harmless. *Aphthous ulcers* are usually small and creamy-white and may be so painful that your child will be reluctant to eat. They are sometimes associated with stress and may come in crops during a particularly anxious time, such as starting school. A *traumatic ulcer* is larger and usually starts as a sore patch on the inside of the cheeks, possibly after injury by biting or by the rubbing of a rough tooth. It enlarges to form a painful yellow crater. It heals very slowly and, regardless of treatment, takes 10–14 days to clear completely. White, painful blisters on the roof of the mouth, on the gums and inside the cheeks can be the result of a primary infection with the **cold sore** virus.

POSSIBLE SYMPTOMS

• Small, creamy-white, painful raised areas anywhere on the tongue, gums or lining of the mouth.
• Large red area with a yellow centre, particularly inside the cheeks.
• White blister-like spots inside the mouth, which can sometimes be accompanied by a fever.
• Loss of appetite because eating is too painful.

IS IT SERIOUS?

Mouth ulcers are only rarely serious, but because they can be painful they sometimes cause loss of appetite and interfere with your child's eating.

WHAT SHOULD I DO FIRST?

1 *If your child complains of a sore mouth or tongue, check to see if there are any areas of soreness.*

2 *If the ulcer is large and is inside the cheek, check for a jagged tooth that might be rubbing the cheek lining.*

3 *If the ulcers resemble white curds, try to wipe them off with a clean handkerchief. If this leaves red, raw patches, the ulcers could be caused by oral* **thrush**.

4 *Smear an antiseptic jelly or glycerine over the ulcers with your fingertip, or give your child some liquid paracetamol to relieve the pain.*

5 *If your bottlefed baby has a traumatic ulcer on the roof of his mouth, check the teat. It may be too hard for your baby's tender mouth.*

SHOULD I CONSULT THE DOCTOR?

Consult your doctor as soon as possible if the ulcers are very painful, or your home treatment doesn't help. Consult your doctor as soon as possible if they are recurrent. If the ulceration is caused by a jagged tooth, take your child to the dentist.

WHAT MIGHT THE DOCTOR DO?

• Your doctor will probably prescribe an anti-inflammatory cream for aphthous ulcers. The cream is not dissolved by saliva and therefore clings to the ulcers and speeds healing.
• If your child suffers from recurrent mouth ulcers, your doctor will refer him to hospital for blood tests to see if there is an underlying cause.

SEE ALSO:
Cold sore, *page 48*
Thrush, *page 121*

GUM BOIL

A gum boil, or dental abscess, is a pus-filled cavity that develops at the root of a decayed tooth. In a primary tooth, a gum boil can damage the underlying permanent tooth if it is left untreated. Gum boils are nearly always very painful as they are in such a confined area and the pain does not always respond to painkillers.

IS IT SERIOUS?

A gum boil should be treated seriously as it causes great discomfort and can result in a lost tooth.

POSSIBLE SYMPTOMS

- Red, inflamed lump on one side of the tooth in the gum.
- Throbbing pain.
- Tenderness and swelling on the affected side of the face.
- Swollen neck glands.
- Pain below the ear on the affected side of the face.

WHAT SHOULD I DO FIRST?

1 Examine the gum around the tooth and if you notice a red lump, gently feel it with your fingertip. It will be soft and spongy because of the underlying collection of pus.

2 Give your child doses of paracetamol to try to relieve the pain. Do not use local anaesthetics such as oil of cloves. These can damage the gum margin, leading to more dental problems.

3 Rinse your child's mouth with a weak salt-water solution to speed the bursting of the boil and to wash away any pus that has seeped out.

4 Apply a covered hot-water bottle to your child's cheek to soothe the pain.

SHOULD I CONSULT THE DOCTOR?

Consult your dentist immediately or take your child to the nearest hospital casualty department.

WHAT MIGHT THE DOCTOR DO?

- The dentist or doctor will drain the pus by either opening the gum or removing the tooth if there is no possibility of saving it. Both will be done under an anaesthetic.
- Your dentist or doctor will prescribe a course of antibiotics to eradicate the infection. Your child may also be prescribed a mouthwash to be used three or four times a day until the wound has healed.

WHAT CAN I DO TO HELP?

- Maintain regular tooth brushing to minimize tooth decay.
- Take your child to the dentist regularly from the age of four.
- Cut down on sweets and sugary foods in your child's diet.

SEE ALSO:
Earache, *page 70*
Toothache, *page 80*

CHAPTER

RESPIRATORY SYSTEM

The respiratory system is the name given to the organs responsible for carrying oxygen from the air to the bloodstream and expelling carbon dioxide, the waste product. When the system malfunctions, therefore, it can affect the air passages, lungs and muscles that control breathing. Diseases of the respiratory system can range from the common and minor, such as coughs and hayfever, to more serious diseases such as bronchitis and asthma. All need careful handling (even coughs can be symptomatic of something else or can lead to other problems) as described in the entries that follow.

DIAGNOSIS GUIDE

Because respiratory ailments vary widely from minor to serious, it is particularly important to be able to spot and treat them quickly. To use this section, look for the symptom most similar to the one your child is suffering from then turn to the relevant entry. See also p. 13 for a list of emergency symptoms.

RUNNY NOSE, WEEPY, RED-RIMMED, ITCHY EYES
possibly **Hayfever**, see p. 89

COUGHING
accompanied by grasping the throat and redness in the face
possibly **Choking**, see p. 92

DRY COUGH
with a fever and rapid, laboured breathing
possibly **Bronchitis**, see p. 86

HOARSE COUGH OR LOSS OF VOICE
possibly **Croup**, see p. 88 or **Laryngitis**, see p. 68

WHOOPING SOUND
during a coughing fit as air is breathed in
possibly **Whooping cough**, see p.93

LABOURED BREATHING
with wheezing and sensation of suffocation
possibly **Asthma**, see p. 90

COUGH

A cough is either a symptom of a disease or the body's way of reacting to an irritant in the throat or air passages. A *wet cough* or *productive cough* may bring up phlegm from the chest and clear mucus from the air passages, for example, during an attack of **asthma** or **whooping cough**. A *dry cough*, which produces no phlegm, does not always have an obvious cause. The irritation provoking the cough may be mucus from chronically infected sinuses or nasal discharge from a common cold, or it may also be the body's way of bringing up a foreign body stuck in the windpipe. If adults smoke a lot around your child, the smoke may irritate his throat and cause a cough. Children can also sometimes adopt a cough as an attention-seeking device.

IS IT SERIOUS?

A cough is not usually serious, although it can be irritating. However, a cough that causes breathing difficulties is serious and should be treated as an emergency.

WHAT SHOULD I DO FIRST?

1 If your child is coughing up phlegm, lay him over your lap as if you were going to spank him. Pat him gently on the back to help him bring up the phlegm.

2 If you think that your child has a foreign body in his throat, see Choking, p 92.

3 If he is coughing at night, prop him up with pillows. This will stop mucus or nasal discharge from dribbling down the throat. To soothe his throat, give him hot lemon sweetened with honey.

SHOULD I CONSULT THE DOCTOR?

Consult your doctor as soon as possible if the cough doesn't get better after three or four days, if your child is not getting any sleep, or if you cannot remove a foreign body from his throat. Consult him if your baby develops a hacking cough or if your child's coughing is accompanied by rapid, laboured or wheezy breathing. This could be **croup** or asthma.

WHAT MIGHT THE DOCTOR DO?

• If your child's cough is part of an infection such as **tonsillitis**, or croup, your doctor will prescribe antibiotics.

• If your child is suffering from a viral infection, your doctor will advise you on how to relieve the symptoms.

• If the cough is part of an asthmatic condition, your doctor may prescribe bronchodilator drugs.

• Your doctor may prescribe nose drops to administer sparingly to your child before he goes to bed. These drops ease congestion and prevent mucus from dribbling down the back of his throat.

• He may prescribe a cough medicine.

WHAT CAN I DO TO HELP?

• Keep your child warm to help prevent any minor infection from spreading into the lungs, but don't overheat the room.

• Keep the air in his room moist by leaving a window open.

• Avoid giving him cough suppressants.

SEE ALSO:
Asthma, *page 90*
Bronchitis, *page 86*
Choking, *page 92*
Common cold, *page 63*
Croup, *page 88*
Tonsillitis, *page 67*
Whooping cough, *page 93*

BRONCHITIS

Bronchitis is inflammation of the membranes that line the airways leading to the lungs. It arises when a minor infection, such as a **common cold,** reduces resistance to infection. The lining of the airways swell and mucus builds up, making breathing difficult. A hacking **cough** produces phlegm which, if the child swallows, may make him vomit.

IS IT SERIOUS?

In children over a year old, bronchitis is not usually serious, but in rare cases it may require hospitalization.

POSSIBLE SYMPTOMS

- Raised temperature.
- Dry, hacking cough, changing to a cough that produces green or yellow phlegm.
- Rapid breathing, over 40 breaths per minute, with wheezing.
- Breathing difficulties.
- Loss of appetite.
- Vomiting with the cough.
- Blueness of the lips and tongue.

WHAT SHOULD I DO FIRST?

1 If your child has recently had a cold, sore throat, sinusitis or an ear infection, and his condition worsens, take his temperature. If he has a fever, take his temperature every four hours. If it is as high as 38°C (100.4°F), lower it by tepid sponging (see p. 26).

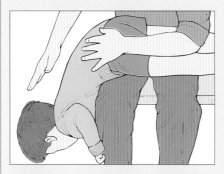

2 If he is coughing, check if there is any phlegm. If there is, encourage him to cough it up. Hold him over your lap if he cannot understand how to do this, and pat him on the back during the coughing attack.

3 Keep offering your child liquids to prevent dehydration. Avoid patent cough suppressants if there is phlegm, as it needs to be coughed up.

SHOULD I CONSULT THE DOCTOR?

Consult your doctor immediately or take your child to the nearest hospital casualty department if he has difficulty breathing, is drawing in his chest with every breath, or if there is any sign of blueness around his lips and on his tongue. This should be treated as an emergency. Always consult your doctor if his infection gets worse.

WHAT MIGHT THE DOCTOR DO?

- If your child is in great distress because of breathing difficulties or vomiting, your doctor may admit him to hospital so that he can be given either oxygen to help with breathing, or intravenous fluids to prevent dehydration.
- Your doctor will prescribe antibiotics if a bacterial infection is present. If your child's bronchitis is caused by a virus, you will be advised on nursing procedures because there is no specific medication.

SEE ALSO:
Common cold, *page 63*
Cough, *page 85*
Sinusitis, *page 65*
Sore throat, *page 66*
Vomiting, *page 100*

INFLUENZA

Influenza ('flu), like the **common cold**, is caused by a virus and has no known cure. It lasts around three to four days. Unless there is a secondary infection, treatment of the symptoms is usually all that is necessary in most cases.

IS IT SERIOUS?

It is rare for serious complications to occur with influenza. However, natural resistance is reduced and a secondary infection, such as pneumonia, **earache**, **bronchitis** or **sinusitis**, could result. Influenza is always serious in a child who has **asthma**, or a condition such as diabetes mellitus.

POSSIBLE SYMPTOMS

- Runny nose.
- Sore throat.
- Cough.
- Temperature above 38°C (100.4°F).
- Shivering.
- Aches and pains.
- Diarrhoea, vomiting or nausea.
- Weakness and lethargy.

WHAT SHOULD I DO FIRST?

1 *Check your child's temperature every 3–4 hours. If it has not come down after 36 hours, call your doctor.*

2 *Give your child paracetamol and put him to bed.*

3 *Don't force your child to eat, but make sure he gets plenty to drink.*

4 *If a rash appears just after the onset of 'flu symptoms, your child may have* **measles** *rather than influenza.*

SHOULD I CONSULT THE DOCTOR?

Consult your doctor immediately if your child's temperature fails to come down within 36 hours, if you notice a deterioration in his condition after 48 hours, or if you suspect measles. Watch out for a worsening cough, which may suggest a chest infection, earache, or yellow pus discharge from the nose, which may indicate sinusitis.

WHAT MIGHT THE DOCTOR DO?

If there is a secondary infection, your doctor will prescribe an antibiotic.

WHAT CAN I DO TO HELP?

- Your child should rest in bed in a warm room. As soon as he feels better, let him get up, but make him rest if his temperature rises again.
- Dispose of used paper handkerchiefs and wash used fabric handkerchiefs in boiling water.
- You might consider protecting your child with an annual influenza vaccine.
- If, after your child should have recovered, his temperature rises and he vomits, consult your doctor immediately. A rare but serious illness, Reye's syndrome, could be the cause.

SEE ALSO:
Asthma, *page 90*
Bronchitis, *page 86*
Common cold, *page 63*
Cough, *page 85*
Earache, *page 70*
Fever, *page 25*
Measles, *page 28*

CROUP

Croup is the name given to the sound made when air is breathed in through a constricted windpipe, past inflamed vocal cords. It usually occurs only in young children up to the age of about four, who are susceptible because their air passages (*bronchi*) are narrow and become blocked with mucus when inflamed – most commonly because of a virus such as a **common cold**, or an infection such as **bronchitis**. In rare cases, croup can be caused by an inhaled **foreign body**. In older children the condition is less serious and is known as **laryngitis**. The first attack of croup can come on quickly, usually at night, and it may last a couple of hours.

POSSIBLE SYMPTOMS

- Croaking cough.
- Laboured breathing when the lower chest caves in at every inhalation.
- Wheezing.
- Face colour becoming grey or blue.

Your child will have a croaking, barking cough and laboured breathing.

IS IT SERIOUS?

If your child has a severe attack of croup, he could develop breathing difficulties. This should be treated as an emergency.

WHAT SHOULD I DO FIRST?

1 Stay calm and try to soothe your child so that he won't panic and make his breathing more difficult.

2 Your child's air passages will be soothed by moist air. If the air outside is cool and damp, take him to the window and get him to take a deep breath of air, or take him into the bathroom and turn on the hot taps to build up a steamy atmosphere.

3 Prop your child up comfortably in bed with pillows or hold him on your lap. It will be easier for him to breathe if he is sitting up.

SHOULD I CONSULT THE DOCTOR?

Consult your doctor immediately if your child's skin turns grey or blue and he has to fight for breath. Consult your doctor as soon as possible to tell him that your child has had an attack of croup.

WHAT MIGHT THE DOCTOR DO?

- In a serious attack, your doctor will give your child oxygen.
- If necessary, your doctor will prescribe antibiotics to eradicate any underlying infection.
- Your doctor will give you advice on what to do should your child have another attack.
- If the attack is caused by an inhaled foreign body, your doctor will remove the foreign body.

WHAT CAN I DO TO HELP?

If any further attacks occur, stay with your child and follow your doctor's instructions.

SEE ALSO:
Bronchitis, *page 86*
Common cold, *page 63*
Laryngitis, *page 68*
Nose, foreign body in, *page 73*

HAYFEVER

Hayfever is similar to **asthma** except that the allergic reaction occurs in the mucous membranes of the nose and eyelids, not in the chest. The condition is also known as allergic rhinitis and causes sneezing, a runny nose and itchy, watery eyes. It occurs in spring and summer and is usually due to a reaction to pollen from flowers, grasses and trees. Most hayfever sufferers are sensitive to more than one pollen and, short of isolation in an air-conditioned room, it is difficult for them to avoid the symptoms. Children who suffer from hayfever can become mouth-breathers because the nose is so blocked. Hayfever tends not to occur before the age of five, but it can start or stop

at any time, and it tends to run in families. Some children who are allergic to animals and house dust as well as pollens, suffer all year round from hayfever; this condition is called perennial allergic rhinitis.

POSSIBLE SYMPTOMS
• Sneezing. • Runny nose with clear discharge. • Itchy, watery, red-rimmed eyes.

IS IT SERIOUS?

Hayfever is periodically troublesome, but it has no serious consequences.

WHAT SHOULD I DO FIRST?

1 If your child is sneezing a lot, check his temperature to make sure he isn't ill with an infection such as **influenza** *or a* **common cold.**

2 Discourage your child from rubbing his eyes; this will make them worse. Bathe his eyes with cool water to ease the irritation.

SHOULD I CONSULT THE DOCTOR?

Consult your doctor as soon as possible if you think your child may be suffering from a more serious infection, or if the hayfever is making him miserable.

WHAT MIGHT THE DOCTOR DO?

• Your doctor will probably prescribe decongestant nasal drops or antihistamine spray, liquid or tablets to relieve the symptoms.
• If your child's condition is severe, your doctor may arrange for him to have a series of skin tests to track down the allergen that is causing the symptoms. Once the allergens have been identified,

a special vaccine can be made for him and a course of desensitizing injections given over a period of weeks to protect him. These don't always work, however, and have to be given during the winter.

WHAT CAN I DO TO HELP?

• Watch the pollen count each day and if it is high, discourage your child from playing near freshly-mown grassland.
• Avoid feathers in your child's bedding and fluff in his clothing.
• Keep your house as dust-free as possible. Even if your child isn't allergic to dust, a dusty atmosphere makes the condition worse.
• Prepare an emergency pack for outings. It should contain paper hand-kerchiefs, eye drops, a moist towel to soothe your child's eyes, and whatever medication has been prescribed.

SEE ALSO:
Asthma, *page 90*
Common cold, *page 63*
Influenza, *page 87*

ASTHMA

Asthma is an allergic disease which affects the air passages (*bronchi*). When the allergic reaction takes place, the bronchi constrict and become clogged with mucus, making breathing difficult. An asthma attack can be very frightening for a young child because the feeling of suffocation can cause panic, making breathing even more difficult. The initial cause of the allergic reaction, the allergen, is usually airborne – pollen or house dust, for example. Once asthma is established, emotional stress and exercise can also bring on an attack.

Asthma does not usually begin until a child is about two years of age. The condition tends to run in families and is unfortunately usually accompanied by other allergic diseases, such as **eczema** or **hayfever**. However, more than half of the children who suffer from asthma eventually grow out of it by early adulthood; in many of the rest, the attacks become less severe as they grow older.

Many babies under one year wheeze if they suffer from bronchiolitis, when their small air passages become inflamed. These babies are not necessarily suffering from asthma; as they grow and their air passages widen, the wheezing will stop. Infection, rather than an allergic reaction, is the usual cause of this.

POSSIBLE SYMPTOMS

- Laboured breathing: breathing out becomes difficult and the abdomen may be drawn inward with the effort of breathing in.
- Sensation of suffocation.
- Wheezing.
- Persistent cough.
- Blueness around the lips (cyanosis) because of lack of oxygen.

AREA AFFECTED

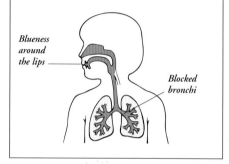

Blueness around the lips

Blocked bronchi

IS IT SERIOUS?

Asthma attacks can be frightening, but with medication and advice from your doctor, your child should suffer no serious complications.

WHAT SHOULD I DO FIRST?

1 Consult your doctor immediately if you have reason to think your child is having an asthma attack.

2 If a bronchodilator medicine has been prescribed for your child, help him use it as instructed.

3 If the attack occurs when your child is in bed, sit him up, propped up with pillows; otherwise, sit him on a chair with his arms braced against the back so that he can take the weight off his chest; this will allow the chest muscles to force air out more efficiently.

4 Stay calm; a show of anxiety from you will only make him more upset. While waiting for the doctor, try to take your child's mind off the asthma attack.

SHOULD I CONSULT THE DOCTOR?

Consult your doctor immediately if your child is having an asthma attack.

ASTHMA

WHAT MIGHT THE DOCTOR DO?

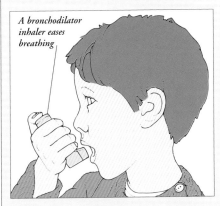

A bronchodilator inhaler eases breathing

• Your doctor will probably treat the attack with a bronchodilator drug, which is inhaled directly into the bronchi and gets right to the site of the restriction. A severe attack may require treatment in hospital, where larger doses of bronchodilator drugs may be given.

• If there is some evidence of a chest infection, antibiotics will be prescribed. Your doctor will measure your child's peak expiry flow rate (PEFR) to monitor his condition.

• Your doctor will discuss prevention of further attacks. He may try to determine the allergen. He will arrange for you to have a small supply of a bronchodilator drug, either in liquid form or as capsules for insertion in an inhaler or spacer. This should be given as soon as an attack begins. Your doctor will ask you to inform him if your child has a severe attack, or if an attack does not respond to two doses of the bronchodilator.

• Your doctor may prescribe a steroid drug if other simpler measures don't prevent further attacks. A small dose of steroid may be inhaled three or four times a day or, if this is not effective, a larger dose will be given in tablet form.

• Your health visitor can help you monitor the severity and frequency of your child's attacks and give general advice about ongoing treatment.

WHAT CAN I DO TO HELP?

• If your doctor failed to pinpoint the allergen, try to track it down yourself. Notice when the attacks occur and at what time of the day or year. Avoid obvious allergens, such as feather pillows, and keep the dust down in your house by vacuuming floors often.

• Many asthmatics are allergic to animals. If you have a pet, ask a friend to look after it for a while and see if your child's attacks are reduced.

• Make sure your child has the prescribed drugs nearby at all times. Inform his school about his asthma.

• Ask to be referred to a physiotherapist so that your child can learn breathing exercises to help him remain calm during an attack.

• Encourage your child to stand and sit up straight so that his lungs have more space. Don't allow him to become overweight as this will put an extra burden on his lungs.

• Moderate exercise can help his breathing, but too much can bring on an asthma attack. Swimming, however, can be especially helpful.

• Avoid smoking near your child.

SEE ALSO:
Eczema, *page 51*
Hayfever, *page 89*

CHOKING

Choking is the way of dislodging a foreign body that has entered the airway instead of the passage to the stomach. If there is enough air getting through to the lungs, the object should be able to be coughed back up into the mouth.

POSSIBLE SYMPTOMS

- Coughing.
- Grasping the throat.
- Redness, followed by blueness in the face – the blood vessels in the neck and face may stand out.

IS IT SERIOUS?

If your child is coughing and gasping for breath, or turning red then blue in the face, this is an emergency and you should call for medical help. If the airway is totally blocked, he will lose consciousness and stop breathing; if this happens, call for help and give mouth-to-mouth ventilation.

WHAT SHOULD I DO FIRST?

If your baby is choking

1 *Lay him along your forearm, with his head lower than his chest and his chin supported between your fingers. Give up to five sharp slaps on the middle of his back with your other hand.*

2 *If the foreign body is coughed into the throat and you can see it, try to hook it out with a finger. Be careful not to push the object further down. Hold your baby steady with your other hand to prevent him from re-inhaling the object.*

3 *If you cannot hook it out give him alternate back slaps and chest thrusts. To do chest thrusts, put two fingers on his lower breastbone, just below the nipple line, and thrust downwards. Check his mouth to see if the obstruction has cleared.*

If your child is choking

1 *Bend him forward with his head lower than his chest. Give him up to five firm back slaps between his shoulders.*

2 *If the foreign body is coughed into the throat and you can see it, try to hook it out very carefully with a finger.*

3 *If you cannot hook it out, give your child alternating back slaps, chest and abdominal thrusts. To do chest thrusts, stand behind him and make a fist with one hand. Curve it round his front, place against his lower breastbone and grasp with your other hand. Press into his chest with a quick inward thrust. For abdominal thrusts, also stand behind him and make a fist with one hand. Curve it round his front and place it against his central upper abdomen. Grasp your fist with your other hand, then press both together into his abdomen in a quick upward thrusting movement. Check his mouth to see if the obstruction has cleared.*

SHOULD I CONSULT THE DOCTOR?

If the obstruction has not cleared and your baby or child turns blue or loses consciousness, call for an ambulance immediately and inform the operator of his condition. If he is conscious, continue giving your baby alternate back slaps and chest thrusts, or your child back slaps, abdominal and chest thrusts while waiting for medical help. If your baby or child loses consciousness or stops breathing, get emergency advice by telephone about what to do until help arrives.

WHOOPING COUGH

Whooping cough is one of the most dangerous childhood diseases, especially in babies under a year old.

It begins as an ordinary cold with a cough. The coughing becomes severe, with spasmodic bouts which make it difficult to breathe. When your child manages to draw breath, there is a "whooping" sound as air is drawn in past the swollen larynx. Breathing difficulties are even greater for babies, who may never develop the technique of whooping to get air into their lungs. Sometimes **vomiting** occurs after a coughing bout. The coughing phase of whooping cough can last for up to 10 weeks. The risk of developing a secondary infection, such as **bronchitis**, is high after this disease.

POSSIBLE SYMPTOMS

- Cold symptoms of a fever, runny nose, aches and pains.
- Excessive coughing, with a characteristic "whoop" as the child struggles to draw breath.
- Vomiting after a coughing bout.
- Sleeplessness because of coughing.

IS IT SERIOUS?

Whooping cough is a serious disease, especially in babies. If vomiting is severe, there is also the danger of dehydration. A severe attack can damage the lungs and cause recurrent bronchial infections.

WHAT SHOULD I DO FIRST?

1 If your child's cold fails to improve and his cough worsens, put him to bed and seek medical help.

2 If you suspect your baby has whooping cough, consult your doctor immediately. If you suspect your child has it, keep him from school until you have seen your doctor.

3 If he is having a long coughing bout, sit him up and hold him so that he is leaning slightly forward. Hold a bowl so that he can spit any phlegm into it. Warm, moist inhalations help.

SHOULD I CONSULT THE DOCTOR?

Consult your doctor immediately if you suspect whooping cough.

WHAT MIGHT THE DOCTOR DO?

- Your doctor may prescribe antibiotics to limit the infectiousness of the child. He may need to take a throat swab from your baby to diagnose whooping cough because babies rarely whoop.
- He will keep a close check on a baby with whooping cough and if it is severe, will probably recommend hospital.
- He will make sure you know how to hold your child during a coughing attack. He may advise you to raise the foot of your baby's cot.

WHAT CAN I DO TO HELP?

- Put bowls everywhere so that your child can spit up phlegm or vomit. If he vomits after coughing, give him small meals and drinks afterwards to help him keep some nourishment down.
- Sleep in the room with him so that he is never alone during a coughing bout.
- If, after it has cleared up, he seems sick and is breathing with difficulty, contact your doctor immediately.
- Don't give him cough medication without your doctor's advice.

SEE ALSO:
Bronchitis, *page 86*
Vomiting, *page 100*

COT DEATH

Sudden infant death syndrome (SIDS), or cot death, is the sudden and often unexplained death of a seemingly healthy baby. There is no single known cause of cot death, although research has shown that some deaths can be the result of an abnormality in the breathing and heart rate. There are several current areas of research, including the development of a baby's temperature control mechanism and respiratory system in the first six months, and the recent discovery that an inherited enzyme deficiency may be responsible for around 1 per cent of cases. Studies connecting SIDS with flame-retardant chemicals in cot mattresses have, so far, proven inconclusive.

The death of an infant from SIDS is a particularly distressing experience. Severe grief can be compounded by intense

POSSIBLE SYMPTOMS
- Common cold-like symptom of stuffy nose.
- Inexplicable weight loss.

feelings of guilt and misplaced blame, and family relationships can sometimes suffer as a result. Parents of cot death infants may have to discuss the incident with the police and be prepared for post-mortem examination of the baby. Your doctor, paediatrician and health visitor should all provide valuable support and counselling in this situation, and talking to other parents who have also experienced a cot death, or to a professional organization, can also provide great comfort.

WHAT CAN I DO TO HELP?

While the causes of cot death are not clear, there are ways in which you can significantly reduce the risks.
- Always put your baby to sleep ON HIS BACK, NEVER ON HIS FRONT. Babies who sleep on their backs are at less risk of cot death. This position also helps control your baby's body temperature (see below).
- Don't wrap him in too many night-clothes or bedclothes, especially during winter, or put him to bed in a room that is too warm. Use a thermostatically-controlled heater in his room so that temperatures do not rise too high or drop too low. Make sure he has enough blankets – a sheet and three blankets is sufficient in a room temperature of 18°C (64°F). Use fewer if the temperature is higher – no more than one sheet and blanket on a warm night of 24°C (75°F).
- Avoid smoking during pregnancy and after your child is born.
- Ban smokers from the house.
- Be careful not to swaddle or tuck your baby in. Don't use baby nests, sheep-skins, duvets and cot bumpers as they all prevent heat loss.
- Whenever possible, breastfeed rather than bottle-feed your baby.
- Avoid taking unnecessary drugs during pregnancy.
- If you think your baby is unwell, contact your doctor. If he has a fever, don't increase the wrapping – reduce it so he can lose heat. After a minor illness, keep a closer eye than usual on him for several days until the symptoms disappear.

FOR HELP AND ADVICE CONTACT:
Foundation for the Study of Infant Death
14 Halkin Street
London SW1X 7DP
0171 235 1721

DIGESTIVE SYSTEM

The digestive system is that part of the body that
directly processes food (the digestive tract) and includes
various associated organs, such as the salivary glands,
liver and pancreas. Together, they are responsible for
absorbing and breaking down food to provide energy
to build and repair cells and tissues. The range of
complaints, symptoms and ailments that can affect the
efficient working of this system include colic, food
poisoning, vomiting and gastroenteritis. All are
described in detail, with practical suggestions as to
how you can help, in the entries that follow.

DIAGNOSIS GUIDE

Because young children are prone to a variety of acute digestive complaints, it is important that you are able to deal with them efficently. To use this section, look for the symptom most similar to the one that your child is suffering from, then turn to the relevant entry. See also p. 13 for a list of emergency symptoms.

YOUR BABY BECOMES RED-FACED AND DRAWS HIS LEGS UP usually in the early evening *possibly* **Colic**, see p. 97

PAIN STARTING AROUND THE NAVEL then moving to the lower right area of the groin in an older child *possibly* **Appendicitis**, see p. 106

PAINLESS BULGE IN THE SKIN'S SURFACE near the navel or in the groin, accompanied by vomiting with sharp abdominal pain *possibly* **Hernia**, see p. 105

LOOSE, FREQUENT BOWEL MOTIONS accompanied by vomiting shortly after eating and possible raised temperature *possibly* **Food poisoning**, see p. 99 or **Gastroenteritis**, see p. 98

HARD, PEBBLE-LIKE STOOLS and pain in the lower abdomen *possibly* **Constipation**, see p. 103

LOOSE, FREQUENT BOWEL MOTIONS *possibly* **Diarrhoea**, see p. 102

COLIC

Colic, as applied to a baby under four months of age, describes a crying spell, during which the baby's face becomes very red and both legs are drawn up to his stomach as if he is in great pain. This crying spell usually comes in the early evening; during the rest of the day the baby is generally contented. The crying can reach screaming pitch and last from one to three hours. It doesn't usually respond to soothing techniques that work at other times. Colic is so common that it is regarded by paediatricians as normal, but for parents it can be difficult to endure. The cause of the apparent spasmodic pain is not known. It is often at its worst at three months of age but disappears by four months.

POSSIBLE SYMPTOMS

• Your baby cannot settle in the early evening and cries no matter what you do to calm him.
• He becomes red-faced and draws his legs up into his stomach as if in pain.
• He may wake from a short sleep with a startled cry.

IS IT SERIOUS?

The fact that your baby is contented during the rest of the day means that this crying bout is not related to a serious physical problem. Colicky babies are usually healthy and thriving.

WHAT SHOULD I DO FIRST?

1 *Try all the methods of soothing your baby that you know work at other times of the day. This may mean you are constantly offering the breast or bottle; changing nappies; winding; nursing and rocking; walking with the baby held over your shoulder; putting the baby in a sling against your body; playing music to give a constant background noise; or walking him in a pram.*

2 *Carefully lay him on his tummy positioned over a hot-water bottle wrapped in a towel.*

3 *Try using a dummy: your baby may need to suck all the time.*

4 *Don't use any patent medicines without your doctor's advice.*

5 *Bathe your baby at this difficult time of the day. A warm bath relaxes most babies and this will pass the time when the crying seems worst.*

SHOULD I CONSULT THE DOCTOR?

Consult your doctor as soon as possible if you find you cannot cope with the nightly crying sessions.

WHAT MIGHT THE DOCTOR DO?

• Your doctor will reassure you that your baby is healthy and that he will grow out of the colic eventually.
• Health visitors can provide valuable advice and counselling while your baby is still having attacks.

WHAT CAN I DO TO HELP?

• Make sure you look after yourself. You will be better able to cope if you get as much sleep as you possibly can during the day while your baby sleeps.
• Invite good friends in to share that time of the evening with you; a relaxed atmosphere may calm both you and your baby.
• Talk to other parents who have had colicky babies. Once you realize that colic attacks do pass, you may find them easier to bear.

GASTROENTERITIS

Gastroenteritis is inflammation of the stomach and intestines. The most common cause in children is the *rotavirus*, which can be inhaled and tends to spread easily through a community. It may also be caused by direct infection of the intestines, usually from contaminated food (**food poisoning**), or by a parasite, when it is sometimes known as dysentery. Gastroenteritis may also be a symptom of another infection, such as **influenza**.

Gastroenteritis in babies is most common in bottlefed babies and is usually the result of poor sterilization of feeding equipment.

POSSIBLE SYMPTOMS

- Vomiting.
- Nausea.
- Diarrhoea.
- Abdominal cramps.
- Loss of appetite.
- Raised temperature.

IS IT SERIOUS?

Gastroenteritis is very serious in children, especially babies, because **vomiting** and **diarrhoea** can rapidly lead to dehydration.

WHAT SHOULD I DO FIRST?

1 Stop all foods and milk and give your child only water in small amounts every 15 minutes.

2 Put your child to bed with a bowl by the bed in case he vomits.

3 Make sure he washes his hands after going to the toilet.

SHOULD I CONSULT THE DOCTOR?

Consult your doctor immediately if your child has diarrhoea and vomiting for more than six hours and you cannot bring them under control with a fluids-only diet.

WHAT MIGHT THE DOCTOR DO?

- Your doctor will probably prescribe a special powder containing glucose and essential minerals to be added to your child's drinks, to replace what has been lost through vomiting and diarrhoea. To avoid dehydration, your child should be given 200 ml (7 fl oz) of water for every kilogram (2 lb) of his body weight in the first 24 hours of diarrhoea and vomiting.

- Your doctor will recommend bed-rest and a liquid diet until the vomiting and diarrhoea have subsided.
- For a bottlefed baby, he may recommend that you replace milk feeds with a glucose solution and give you a regime for reintroducing formula feeds.
- If your baby is seriously ill, your doctor may admit him to hospital.

WHAT CAN I DO TO HELP?

- Be meticulous about hygiene.
- Avoid giving your child acidic drinks such as orange juice. They may irritate the stomach further.
- Reintroduce foods slowly when he seems interested, starting with easily digested foods such as jellies, yoghurt, soups and non-fatty foods.
- If he refuses to drink enough fluids, or doesn't like the taste of the special glucose powder, give him cubes of melon.

SEE ALSO:
Diarrhoea, *page 102*
Food poisoning, *page 99*
Influenza, *page 87*
Vomiting, *page100*

FOOD POISONING

Food poisoning is a form of **gastroenteritis** caused by eating food contaminated with poisons, usually from bacteria. It usually occurs within three to 24 hours after eating, depending on the poison. *E. coli* is the bacterium most commonly responsible for food poisoning among babies, usually in bottlefed babies; *salmonella* and *staphylococcii* bacteria are also fairly common. Food poisoning symptoms can also arise from eating chemicals, insecticides or even certain plants.

POSSIBLE SYMPTOMS

- Abdominal cramps.
- Fever or vomiting.
- Frequent, loose stools that may contain blood, pus or mucus.
- Muscular weakness and chills.

IS IT SERIOUS?

In a baby, this condition is serious because it can rapidly lead to dehydration.

WHAT SHOULD I DO FIRST?

*1 If your child is **vomiting** and has **diarrhoea**, check his temperature to see if he has a fever. Check his stools for mucus or blood.*

2 Put him to bed and stop all foods, but keep offering him frequent small drinks of water with a pinch of salt and 5ml (1 teaspoonful) of glucose added.

3 Try to determine what could have caused the symptoms.

SHOULD I CONSULT THE DOCTOR?

Consult your doctor immediately if vomiting and diarrhoea continue for more than six hours and you cannot bring them under control with a fluids-only diet. Consult him immediately if your child's condition has not improved within 24 hours, or if you suspect that he has drunk an insecticide or eaten a poisonous plant. If your doctor is delayed, take your child to the nearest casualty department, with the suspected poison.

WHAT MIGHT THE DOCTOR DO?

- In the majority of cases there is no special treatment for food poisoning except to replace fluid and salts lost through diarrhoea and vomiting. Your doctor will probably prescribe a powder containing glucose and essential salts to be added to your child's drinks, and to replace all milk feeds in a bottlefed baby.
- If your child is in danger of dehydration, your doctor will admit him to hospital. If vomiting is severe, he may give him an injection of an anti-emetic drug.

WHAT CAN I DO TO HELP?

- Place a bowl next to your child's bed for him to vomit into, so that he doesn't have to run to the toilet.
- Keep him cool with an icepack or a damp facecloth if he has a fever.
- Help your child rinse his mouth out with water after he has vomited.
- Reintroduce foods that are easily digested, like soups, yoghurt and jellies.
- Be meticulous about hygiene.
- To prevent food poisoning, defrost foods well before cooking, refrigerate all cooked food and reheat it thoroughly.

SEE ALSO:
Diarrhoea, *page 102*
Fever, *page 25*
Gastroenteritis, *page 98*
Vomiting, *page 100*

VOMITING

Consult your doctor immediately if your child continues to vomit over a six-hour period; if vomiting is accompanied by **diarrhoea** or a **fever**; or if the vomiting is accompanied by any other symptoms such as **earache**.

ACCOMPANYING SYMPTOMS	COMMON CAUSES
Your baby often brings up a little milk during or after a feed, but seems contented, feeds well and is gaining weight.	This regurgitation of a little milk – possetting – is normal and harmless.
Your baby is hungry and seems well, but vomits during, or immediately after, his feed.	Solids given before he can chew properly may be the cause. Until your baby is six or seven months old, give puréed foods.
Your baby has a runny or blocked nose, snuffly breathing or a cough.	A **Common cold**, p. 63, can make your baby vomit if he swallows a lot of the mucus it produces. A **Cough**, p. 85, may also make him vomit.
Your bottlefed or weaned baby, or child, seems unwell and has passed frequent, watery stools.	CONSULT YOUR DOCTOR IMMEDIATELY Your baby may have **Gastroenteritis**, p. 98. An older child may have **Food poisoning**, p. 99.
Your child seems unwell, looks flushed and feels hot.	An infection is the most likely cause. See **Fever**, p. 25.
When travelling, your child seems pale and quiet and complains of nausea.	Travel sickness is the most likely cause.
Your child complains of a severe headache on one side of his forehead.	He could have **Migraine**, p. 117.
Your child has abdominal pain around the navel and to the lower right side of his groin.	CONSULT YOUR DOCTOR IMMEDIATELY Your child could have **Appendicitis**, p. 106.
Your baby is in severe pain and is passing stools that contain blood and mucus resembling redcurrant jelly.	CONSULT YOUR DOCTOR IMMEDIATELY Your baby could have a bowel blockage known as intussusception.
Your child cannot bend his neck forward without pain, and turns away from bright light.	CONSULT YOUR DOCTOR IMMEDIATELY Your child may have **Meningitis**, p. 118.

VOMITING

Vomiting is the violent expulsion of the contents of the stomach through the mouth. A baby may posset up small quantities of curdled milk after a feed, but this is normal and harmless and should not be confused with vomiting. Vomiting has many causes (see p. 100), but in the majority of cases there is little warning and after a single bout your child should be comfortable and back to normal again. Vomiting can be a symptom of a specific disorder of the stomach such as pyloric stenosis, or a symptom of an infection, such as an ear infection. It frequently accompanies a **fever**, and even the **common cold** can cause vomiting if your child swallows enough nasal discharge to irritate his stomach. If your child has a bad cough, this can also sometimes cause him to vomit up food that he has recently eaten. Other possible causes of vomiting include **appendicitis**, **meningitis**, **migraine**, **headaches**, **food poisoning** and travel sickness. Children can also occasionally vomit due to excitement and anticipation, although this is generally limited to young toddlers.

IS IT SERIOUS?

Vomiting should always be taken seriously because it can rapidly cause dehydration, particularly in a baby or young child.

WHAT SHOULD I DO FIRST?

1 *Put your child to bed and place a bowl for him to vomit into within easy reach.*

2 *Give your child frequent, small amounts of liquid – preferably cold water with a pinch of salt and 5ml (1 teaspoonful) of glucose added – to prevent dehydration, every 10–15 minutes.*

3 *Check your child's temperature to see if he has a fever too. Keep him cool by wiping his face with a cool, damp cloth.*

4 *Have him brush his teeth to take away the taste.*

SHOULD I CONSULT THE DOCTOR?

Consult your doctor immediately if your child continues to vomit over a six-hour period. Consult him immediately if the vomiting is accompanied by **diarrhoea** or a **fever** over 38°C (100.4°F), or if the vomiting is accompanied by any other worrying symptoms such as **earache**.

WHAT MIGHT THE DOCTOR DO?

• Your doctor will diagnose the cause of the vomiting and will treat your child accordingly. He will also make sure that there is no danger of dehydration.
• Your child may be admitted to hospital to be given fluids intravenously if he is in danger of becoming dehydrated.

WHAT CAN I DO TO HELP?

• Give your child plenty of his favourite drinks, but avoid orange juice and other acidic juices and don't give him milk.
• Feed your child bland foods when the nausea and vomiting have passed. Reintroduce solid foods slowly.

SEE ALSO:
Appendicitis, *page 106*
Common cold, *page 63*
Diarrhoea, *page 102*
Earache, *page 70*
Fever, *page 25*
Food poisoning, *page 99*
Headache, *page 116*
Meningitis, *page 118*
Migraine, *page 117*

DIARRHOEA

Diarrhoea is the frequent passage of loose, watery stools and is a sign of irritation of the intestines.

Once babies begin to take solid foods, bowel motions become firmer and more regular. Loose, frequent stools can result when a baby or child eats too much of a food that is rich in dietary fibre, such as fruit, or they may be a symptom of an infection. Food may have been contaminated with bacteria (**food poisoning**) or an infection from contaminated stools may have been spread to the mouth by unwashed hands. Diarrhoea can also be the symptom of a non-intestinal infection, such as **influenza**, when it may be accompanied by **fever**.

Ironically, stools similar to those of diarrhoea may be caused by constipation. If an older child soils himself with liquid stools, this may be because of a type of constipation known as **encopresis**.

IS IT SERIOUS?

Diarrhoea in a baby is always serious because of the dangers of dehydration. Diarrhoea accompanied by vomiting in a young child is also serious for the same reason, especially if it is accompanied by fever and sweating. Diarrhoea in which the stools are greasy and foul-smelling can be a symptom of a more serious long-term condition, such as cystic fibrosis.

WHAT SHOULD I DO FIRST?

1 *If your baby is under one year old and has had diarrhoea for six hours, consult your doctor immediately.*

2 *Don't give an older child any food or milk, but give frequent drinks of diluted fruit juice or water with a pinch of salt and 5ml (1 teaspoonful) of glucose added.*

3 *Check your child's temperature to see if he has a fever. Reduce any fever with tepid sponging (see p. 26).*

4 *Pay close attention to hygiene. The infection could spread throughout the family if your child doesn't wash his hands after going to the toilet or if you don't wash yours after changing his nappies.*

SHOULD I CONSULT THE DOCTOR?

Consult your doctor immediately if your child has diarrhoea with fever and **vomiting**, or if he still has diarrhoea after 12 hours, or if the stools are greasy or contain mucus or blood.

WHAT MIGHT THE DOCTOR DO?

• Your doctor may prescribe a powder containing glucose and essential salts to be added to drinks. He will recommend bed-rest and a liquid diet until any fever has passed. As a rough guide, your child should drink at least 200ml (7 fl oz) of liquid per kilogram (2 lb) body weight in 24 hours while he has diarrhoea.

• For a bottlefed baby, he will probably suggest that you replace milk feeds with glucose and salt solution, then slowly reintroduce milk. If your baby is breastfed, you will be advised to continue breastfeeding.

WHAT CAN I DO TO HELP?

• Be meticulous about hygiene.
• When the diarrhoea has cleared up, introduce bland foods such as yoghurt.

SEE ALSO:

Encopresis, *page 104*
Fever, *page 25*
Food poisoning, *page 99*
Influenza, *page 87*
Vomiting, *page 100*

CONSTIPATION

Constipation is a word used to describe the consistency of stools, not the regularity or frequency of bowel movements. During babyhood, constipation is unlikely for either breastfed or bottlefed babies. When they start on solid food, however, they can suffer from it if their diet doesn't contain enough fresh fruit, vegetables and liquids. Even if his stools are hard and dry when, because of illness, he is feverish or has been vomiting, this is not true constipation. The body compensates for loss of fluid from vomiting or fever by absorbing water from the stools, and bowel activity should return to normal when the illness has passed.

POSSIBLE SYMPTOMS

- Hard pebble-like stools.
- Pain in the lower abdomen.
- Blood on nappy or underpants.

IS IT SERIOUS?

Occasional constipation is not serious and can be avoided by means of a diet rich in fibre. Chronic constipation can be serious because it can cause problems in later life. Blood in the stools may indicate an underlying disorder and should always be cause for concern.

WHAT SHOULD I DO FIRST?

1 If your child strains when passing stools and complains of pain, check the consistency of what he has passed.

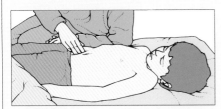

2 If your child complains of stomach pain and it is worse on the right side of his abdomen, check below his navel for possible **appendicitis.**

SHOULD I CONSULT THE DOCTOR?

Consult your doctor immediately if your child complains of pain when moving his bowels. Consult him immediately if you notice blood on your child's nappy or underpants – the passing of a large, dry stool may have injured his anal passage, a complaint that is called anal fissure. Consult your doctor immediately if you suspect he has appendicitis.

WHAT MIGHT THE DOCTOR DO?

- Your doctor may prescribe a mild laxative that is safe to give your child for short periods.
- If your doctor suspects an anal fissure, he will examine your child's rectum, and if there is a tiny crack he will gently lubricate the anal passage to help the skin to heal.

WHAT CAN I DO TO HELP?

- Never give your child laxatives unless your doctor advises it.
- Include as many natural, unprocessed foods as possible in his diet, with some fibre in the form of whole grains – such as wholemeal bread – and fresh fruit and vegetables. It is not a good idea just to scatter bran over your child's meals; this can deplete certain minerals in the diet. A few stewed prunes or dried figs, however, can produce a soft stool within 24 hours.
- Make sure he is getting plenty to drink.

SEE ALSO:
Appendicitis, *page 106*
Encopresis, *page 104*

ENCOPRESIS

If a child frequently soils his underpants after he has been toilet-trained, he is suffering from encopresis. In a child of four or five, uncontrollable bowel motions should be regarded as a symptom of a problem rather than of slow development. The most common cause of encopresis is chronic **constipation**, in which hard, dry stools accumulate in the bowel and loose, watery motions trickle out past them. You may even mistake this condition for **diarrhoea**. The problem often starts as the result of some emotional disturbance in the child's life, such as the arrival of a new baby.

POSSIBLE SYMTOMS

- Involuntary bowel motions after the child has been toilet trained.
- Chronic constipation.

Occasionally, children persist in soiling their pants from infancy onwards. This soiling may be a reaction against over-fussy toilet training.

IS IT SERIOUS?

Encopresis is not a serious problem.

WHAT SHOULD I DO FIRST?

1 Try to determine whether your child is constipated. Ask him when he last went to the toilet.

2 Check whether your child is affected by stress caused by a new baby, moving house or starting school.

SHOULD I CONSULT THE DOCTOR?

Consult your doctor as soon as possible if you think your child has chronic constipation. If you can find no reason for the involuntary soiling, your doctor may be the best person to discover a possible cause of tension.

WHAT MIGHT THE DOCTOR DO?

- If your child is constipated, your doctor will prescribe a mild laxative, specially formulated for babies and children, which is safe for short-term use.

- Your doctor or health visitor will advise you on how to reduce the constipation in the future.
- If there is some emotional reason for the encopresis, your doctor will assess the situation after discussion with you and your child. If he feels that further investigation is needed, your doctor or health visitor may refer you and your child to a psychotherapist.

WHAT CAN I DO TO HELP?

- Make sure your child has a diet rich in dietary fibre and liquids.
- Don't punish your child or show disgust if he soils his pants; this will make the condition worse.
- Watch for signs of poor school performance. Your child may become a target of scorn because of the odour if he soils himself at school. Provide him with spare underpants.

SEE ALSO:
Constipation, *page 103*
Diarrhoea, *page 102*

HERNIA

A hernia results when a small defect in the muscular wall of the abdomen allows soft tissue to protrude through. This appears as a slight bulge in the skin and can be seen even more clearly if your child coughs or strains. The most common type of hernia in children is *umbilical hernia*. This appears near the navel and results from a weakness that occurs in the abdominal wall at birth. An *inguinal hernia* appears lower down in the groin and is most common in boys, the defect occurring after the testicles have descended into the scrotum. Umbilical hernias rarely need any treatment and heal themselves spontaneously. Inguinal hernias may also heal without treatment, but if a small part of the bowel becomes trapped in the hernia it will have to be corrected by minor surgery.

IS IT SERIOUS?

A hernia is not usually serious unless the bowel is trapped.

POSSIBLE SYMPTOMS

- Vomiting with sharp abdominal pain if the bowel has become trapped.
- Painless bulge in the skin's surface near the navel or in the groin; the bulge increases in size when the child coughs, sneezes or cries.

AREAS AFFECTED

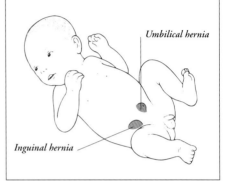

Umbilical hernia

Inguinal hernia

WHAT SHOULD I DO FIRST?

Try to push the hernia carefully inwards. Most hernias respond to gentle pressure by sliding back inside the muscular wall.

SHOULD I CONSULT THE DOCTOR?

Consult your doctor immediately if you notice a bulge in your baby's abdomen before he is six months old. Consult him immediately if a hernia becomes hard, the bulge won't go back with the application of gentle pressure, and there is accompanying abdominal pain and vomiting.

WHAT MIGHT THE DOCTOR DO?

If the hernia is hard or won't go back, your doctor will refer you to a paediatric specialist as it will probably have to be repaired surgically. The operation for a hernia repair is simple. If your child has an inguinal hernia, your doctor may recommend surgical repair to avoid any trapping of the bowel.

WHAT CAN I DO TO HELP?

- Check an umbilical hernia regularly, at bathtimes, for example, to make sure that the hernia is not enlarging, that it is not hard and that it goes back when gently pushed.
- Discuss future action with your doctor and decide together whether to let the hernia heal spontaneously or whether surgery is necessary.
- Take your child for regular check-ups, as directed by your doctor.

APPENDICITIS

Appendicitis occurs when the appendix becomes partly or wholly blocked and a build-up of bacteria causes an infection. The appendix then becomes inflamed and swollen and may need to be removed surgically. An appendicectomy is a common emergency operation among children. However, appendicitis in babies under the age of 12 months is rare.

IS IT SERIOUS?

If appendicitis is diagnosed early, it is not a serious condition. However, if treatment is delayed for any reason, the build-up of pus in the blocked appendix can cause it to burst. This condition is known as peritonitis, and requires immediate attention.

POSSIBLE SYMPTOMS

• Abdominal pain, starting around the navel, then moving down to the lower right abdomen.
• Slight temperature, rarely above 38°C (100.4°F).
• Loss of appetite.
• Vomiting, diarrhoea or constipation.

WHAT SHOULD I DO FIRST?

Check abdomen for tenderness

1 *If your child complains of an abdominal pain for more than a couple of hours, carefully lay him flat on his back. Gently press his stomach a few centimetres to the right of, and just below, the navel. If he experiences any pain on this gentle pressure, and a sharp pain when you suddenly remove your hands, these could both be signs of appendicitis. Consult your doctor immediately.*

2 *If your child is constipated and you suspect appendicitis, don't give him laxatives; they can cause an inflamed appendix to burst.*

3 *Don't give your child anything to eat or drink in case an appendicectomy is necessary.*

SHOULD I CONSULT THE DOCTOR?

Consult your doctor immediately. Any delay could allow the infection to spread to the rest of the intestines.

WHAT MIGHT THE DOCTOR DO?

Your doctor will examine your child's abdomen and ask you to describe symptoms. He will probably arrange for your child to be admitted to hospital to confirm the diagnosis and for surgical removal of the appendix, if necessary.

WHAT CAN I DO TO HELP?

• Arrange to stay with your child at the hospital overnight.
• Encourage your child to rest and eat normally when he returns home from hospital, usually about five days after the operation. Your child should recover fully after two to three weeks.

SEE ALSO:
Constipation, *page 103*

MUSCLES, BONES AND JOINTS

In growing children, the muscles, bones and joints are still developing and are therefore particularly vulnerable to injury. Complaints such as sprains, limps and broken bones may be relatively minor in themselves, but anything that affects the efficient functioning of these parts of the body needs to be taken care of promptly. The entries that follow, therefore, concentrate on recognizing symptoms and show you how to deal with them yourself – and when to consult a doctor.

DIAGNOSIS GUIDE

Most muscle, bone and joint problems in young children are easily spotted. Some, however, are difficult to diagnose accurately. If in doubt always consult your doctor. To use this section, look for the symptom most similar to the one your child is suffering from then turn to the relevant entry. See also p. 13 for a list of emergency symptoms.

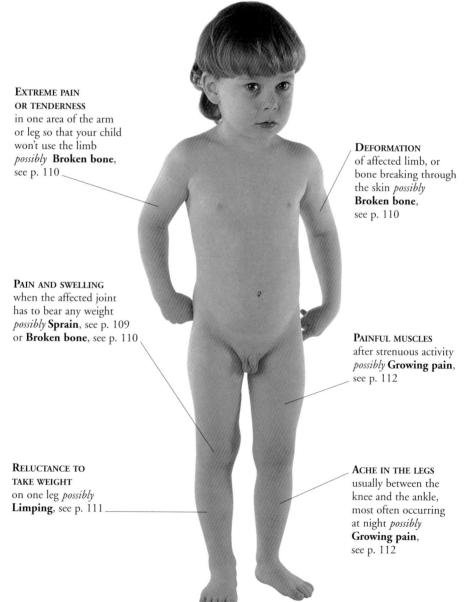

EXTREME PAIN OR TENDERNESS
in one area of the arm or leg so that your child won't use the limb *possibly* **Broken bone**, see p. 110

DEFORMATION
of affected limb, or bone breaking through the skin *possibly* **Broken bone**, see p. 110

PAIN AND SWELLING
when the affected joint has to bear any weight *possibly* **Sprain**, see p. 109 or **Broken bone**, see p. 110

PAINFUL MUSCLES
after strenuous activity *possibly* **Growing pain**, see p. 112

RELUCTANCE TO TAKE WEIGHT
on one leg *possibly* **Limping**, see p. 111

ACHE IN THE LEGS
usually between the knee and the ankle, most often occurring at night *possibly* **Growing pain**, see p. 112

SPRAIN

A sprain is the tearing of the tough, strap-like structures (ligaments) that support a joint and limit its movement. The sprain usually occurs because of overstretching or a sudden twisting action that wrenches the joint beyond its normal movement. The tearing causes bleeding into the joint, which results in swelling, pain and a bad bruise. (If only a few fibres of a ligament tear, it is known as a strain.)

The most common sites of a sprain are the ankle, knee and wrist. Because the ligaments are near the skin's surface in these joints, swelling shows rapidly and your child will not be able to take any weight on the sprained joint.

It is rare for young children to suffer a sprain because their joints are so supple. Sprains are, however, quite common in the six to 12 age group.

IS IT SERIOUS?

A sprain can be painful but it is not serious. Because it can be be difficult to determine without an X-ray whether the injury is a

---

POSSIBLE SYMPTOMS

• Swelling and tenderness.
• Pain when the affected joint has to bear any weight.
• Bruising.

COMMON SITE
OF SPRAIN

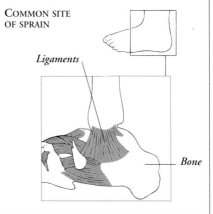

Ligaments

Bone

---

sprain, a **broken bone** or a dislocated joint, it is always sensible to seek medical help if you are not sure.

WHAT SHOULD I DO FIRST?

1 If the affected joint or limb is not misshapen, lay your child down and raise the injured part (if it is misshapen, this could indicate a dislocation or fracture and you should call the doctor).

2 Apply a cold compress to reduce the swelling.

3 Support the joint with a firm crepe bandage applied over a thick wad of cotton wool. Check the bandage regularly to make sure that subsequent swelling has not made it too tight.

4 Encourage your child to rest the joint for at least 24 hours.

SHOULD I CONSULT THE DOCTOR?

Consult your doctor immediately if there is intense pain and the affected joint or limb is misshapen. Consult him as soon as possible if, after 48 hours, the swelling has not subsided or if your child still complains of severe pain and cannot bear any weight on the injured part.

WHAT MIGHT THE DOCTOR DO?

• If your doctor suspects a dislocation or fracture, your child will be referred to a hospital casualty department.
• If the injury is a sprain, your doctor will strap the damaged joint.

SEE ALSO:
Broken bone, *page 110*

Broken Bone

Children's bones do not break as easily as the harder bones of an adult. The most common fracture in children is the *greenstick fracture*, where the bone bends rather than breaks, and where there is minimal damage to the surrounding tissue. In a *simple fracture*, the bone breaks in one place and does not break the skin. In an *open fracture*, the bone ends stick through the skin and may damage blood vessels and muscles.

POSSIBLE SYMPTOMS

• Swelling and bruising around the site of the injury.
• Possible deformation of the affected area.
• Inability to move the affected area normally.
• Pain.

IS IT SERIOUS?

Any type of broken bone, should always be seen and treated promptly by a doctor for a variety of reasons. It has to be set correctly, and any damage to surrounding organs or tissues has to be repaired. There is also risk of infection if the break is an *open fracture* and the bone is exposed to the air.

WHAT SHOULD I DO FIRST?

1 Call an ambulance if the injury involves your child's leg or elbow. Otherwise, take your child to hospital.

2 If the limb appears bent or curved, don't try to straighten it. Don't move your child unless you have to. If a bone has broken through the skin, or if there is a wound leading down to the fracture, drape a sterile dressing over it. Don't attempt any cleaning and don't touch the wound.

3 If there is no bone sticking through the skin, but he cannot move the affected area without pain, immobilize above and below the break: put an arm in a sling; for a leg, tie the knees and ankles together. Take him to the nearest hospital, but call an ambulance if the legs or elbows are affected because you will need a stretcher.

4 Don't give your child anything to eat and drink in case he needs surgery.

5 Keep him warm and calm while you get medical help. Try to raise the affected part after immobilizing it.

SHOULD I CONSULT THE DOCTOR?

Call an ambulance if the bone is bent or curved, if it is sticking through the skin or if a leg or elbow is broken. Take your child to the nearest casualty department if you suspect he has a broken bone.

WHAT MIGHT THE DOCTOR DO?

• The hospital doctor will X-ray your child to determine the extent of the damage. With a straightforward break, the bone will be immobilized by strapping with a tight bandage, or by setting it in a plaster of Paris cast.
• If the break is an open fracture, the bones will be manipulated into position under a general anaesthetic before being immobilized in plaster.
• If there is an open wound with the broken bone, antibiotics will be given.
• If he has a bad break in his leg, he may have to remain in hospital in traction.

WHAT CAN I DO TO HELP?

If your child has a plaster cast, make sure it stays dry. Most broken bones in children heal within six to ten weeks, depending on the severity of the fracture.

LIMPING

Your child is limping if he is not taking the full weight of his body on one leg as he walks. The cause may be obvious, such as a **cut**, a **blister** or a **splinter** on the sole of the foot, an **ingrowing toenail**, a pebble in a shoe or tight shoes.

IS IT SERIOUS?

A persistent limp that seems to have no apparent reason should always be treated seriously in a child since it may be a symptom of a more serious problem. You should always consult your doctor if your child limps. An unexplained limp can be a symptom of the rare form of blood cancer, leukaemia. If the limp is accompanied by any swelling or tenderness of the joints, this could be caused by rheumatic fever, arthritis or osteomyelitis. All of these diseases could have long-term complications and should therefore be treated seriously.

WHAT SHOULD I DO FIRST?

1 Look for obvious injuries and examine any areas that your child claims are painful.

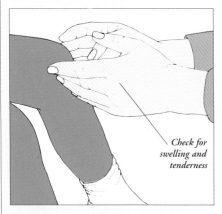

Check for swelling and tenderness

2 Check to see if the joints are swollen and inflamed.

*3 If you suspect your child may have a **broken bone** in his foot or toe, don't hesitate to get medical attention; if the bone is in his leg, call an ambulance. The injury may not always be obvious.*

SHOULD I CONSULT THE DOCTOR?

Consult your doctor immediately for a thorough examination of the limp if you can't find a reason for it, or if you suspect a broken bone. Consult your doctor immediately if any of your child's joints are swollen or tender.

WHAT MIGHT THE DOCTOR DO?

• Your doctor will examine your child's leg thoroughly and may refer him to a paediatric orthopaedic surgeon to find the cause of the problem.
• If a bone in your child's leg is broken, your doctor will refer him to the nearest hospital for an X-ray and to have the leg put into plaster.

WHAT CAN I DO TO HELP?

Never give up if your child has an unexplained limp. Continue taking your child to your doctor so that he can investigate possible causes, and be persistent until the cause is identified.

SEE ALSO:
Blister, *page 41*
Broken bone, *page 110*
Cuts and grazes, *page 36*
Ingrowing toenail, *page 59*

GROWING PAIN

A growing pain is a dull, vague ache in a limb; it doesn't last long and the child can usually be distracted from it. One in six children of school age suffers from some kind of growing pain. Such pains can occur when your child is going through a growth spurt; the muscles and bones grow at slightly different rates, leading to an aching soreness that is worse in the evening. Growing pains can also occur after strenuous activity. It is important to distinguish a growing pain from joint pain. A growing pain is felt between the joints of a limb; joint pain is specific to the joint area. In a child, a joint pain can also be a symptom of rheumatic fever or arthritis.

POSSIBLE SYMPTOMS

- Aches and pains in the arms or legs, most often in the legs.
- Disturbed sleep if the pain is severe.
- Painful muscles after strenuous activity.

IS IT SERIOUS?

A growing pain is not serious, but any pain in the joint could be, particularly if it is accompanied by a **fever**. This could be septic arthritis. You should consult your doctor as soon as possible if your child has these symptoms.

WHAT SHOULD I DO FIRST?

1 *Check your child's joints for swelling and tenderness by pressing on and around them. If there is neither, check the muscles in the same way.*

2 *Check to see if your child limps when he walks.*

3 *Ask your child when the pain started and how long it lasts.*

SHOULD I CONSULT THE DOCTOR?

Consult your doctor as soon as possible if the pain is sited around a joint and is accompanied by a fever, or if it lasts longer than 24 hours.

WHAT MIGHT THE DOCTOR DO?

After excluding any other possible causes of the pain, your doctor will reassure you and your child that there is no cause for you to be concerned.

WHAT CAN I DO TO HELP?

- Show sympathetic interest in the pain – this may be sufficient to relax your child.
- Give your child a warm bath before going to bed or a hot-water bottle to take to bed: both of these can be very soothing if your child is having difficulty sleeping.
- Gently massage the affected muscles to relax any tension.

SEE ALSO:
Fever, *page 25*
Limping, *page 111*

NERVOUS SYSTEM

The nervous system is the body's information-gathering and control mechanism. It is made up of the brain and the spinal cord, and consists of millions of interconnecting nerve cells. Diseases and disorders of the nervous system that are most likely to affect children include dizziness, headache, migraine and, most serious of all, meningitis. Background information on all of these conditions is given in this chapter, together with comprehensive self-help advice and information on when it is necessary to seek medical assistance.

DIAGNOSIS GUIDE

Children find it difficult to describe pain; they may simply appear "ill". A hand held to the head may signify a headache, so never hesitate to contact your doctor for clarification. Check your baby's temperature – any headache plus fever is serious. To use this section, look for the signs most similar to the ones that your child has, then turn to the relevant entry. See also p. 13 for a list of emergency symptoms.

HEADACHE
on one side of the forehead, usually accompanied by vomiting and abdominal pain *possibly* **Migraine**, see p. 117

HEADACHE
accompanied by throbbing in the cheek *possibly* **Gum boil**, see p. 82

STIFF NECK
accompanied by headache *possibly* **Meningitis**, see p. 118

PURPLE-RED RASH
and inability to tolerate bright light *possibly* **Meningitis**, see p. 118

BULGING FONTANELLE
in a baby under the age of 18 months *possibly* **Meningitis**, see p. 118

INTOLERANCE OF BRIGHT LIGHT
accompanied by fever and headache *possibly* **Meningitis**, see p. 118

INTENSE HEADACHE
when the head moves, accompanied by slight fever and blocked nose *possibly* **Sinusitis**, see p. 65

VOMITING AND ABDOMINAL PAIN
accompanied by headache *possibly* **Migraine**, see p. 117

DIZZINESS

Dizziness describes a feeling of unsteadiness and spinning about. When a child is out of breath, he may feel a bit dizzy because there is a less than normal supply of oxygen to his brain. Your child may also feel dizzy if he is suffering from anaemia. A bang on the head that results in loss of consciousness, or a convulsion, may be preceded by dizziness.

However, under normal circumstances, dizziness should usually clear up within two or three minutes.

IS IT SERIOUS?

Momentary dizziness is not serious, but if dizzy spells last longer than 12 hours, they may be caused by anaemia.

WHAT SHOULD I DO FIRST?

1 *Lay your child down and prop his legs up on some cushions. This increases the flow of blood, and therefore oxygen, to his brain. Loosen any tight clothing and tell him to take a few deep breaths.*

2 *Keep him quiet and calm if that is what he wants.*

3 *Note how long he says the dizzy feeling lasts.*

SHOULD I CONSULT THE DOCTOR?

Consult your doctor immediately if your child experiences dizzy spells over a 12-hour period but has no other symptoms. Consult your doctor as soon as possible if your child is continually complaining of dizziness after strenuous activity; this may be a sign of anaemia.

WHAT MIGHT THE DOCTOR DO?

After examining your child, your doctor will determine the cause of the dizziness. If the dizziness is a symptom of a more serious disorder, such as anaemia, your doctor will treat this accordingly.

HEADACHE

About one in five children suffers from recurrent headaches, although a serious physical cause is hardly ever found. Most commonly children complain of pain in their heads after sitting in a hot, stuffy room, if they are worried or anxious about something, if they have a **fever**, or they have **sinusitis** or **toothache**, for example. Some children complain frequently of headache and stomach ache. Such pain is known as abdominal **migraine**. If your child has had a recent injury to his head, and continues to have headaches, you should get immediate medical attention.

IS IT SERIOUS?

Headaches are rarely serious, but if a single headache is accompanied by a fever, neck stiffness, confusion or an intolerance of bright light, this may be a symptom of a more serious illness, such as **meningitis**, and you should seek medical advice.

WHAT SHOULD I DO FIRST?

*1 Ask your child if he has pain anywhere else. Run your hands over the area around his cheeks, jaw and ears to see if sinusitis, a **gum boil**, toothache or **earache** are the problem.*

*2 Check his temperature to see if he has a fever. Headache and fever could be among the first symptoms of an infectious illness such as **measles** or **influenza**.*

3 Check to see if your child has any injury to his head.

4 If the headaches are frequent, find out if your child is worried about anything, such as his school work.

5 If he complains of nausea or vomits, this could be a migraine headache.

6 If he has no other symptoms to concern you, give him a dose of paracetamol to relieve the pain, and put him to bed in a darkened room for half an hour.

SHOULD I CONSULT THE DOCTOR?

Consult your doctor immediately if the headache is accompanied by a temperature of 38°C (100.4°F) with **vomiting**, neck stiffness and intolerance of bright light, or if your child has had a recent head injury. Consult him as soon as possible if headaches are persistent.

WHAT MIGHT THE DOCTOR DO?

• Your doctor will examine your child. This may include taking your child's blood pressure and looking at the retina in the eye. Further tests will be carried out only if your doctor finds something wrong apart from the headaches.
• If the headache is a symptom of a more serious condition, your doctor will treat the condition accordingly.

WHAT CAN I DO TO HELP?

If your child complains of headaches at the end of a school day, give him a drink and a nutritious snack, and encourage him to go out and play in the fresh air.

SEE ALSO:
Earache, *page 70*
Fever, *page 25*
Gum boil, *page 82*
Influenza, *page 87*
Measles, *page 28*
Meningitis, *page 118*
Migraine, *page 117*
Sinusitis, *page 65*
Toothache, *page 80*

MIGRAINE

Migraine is a severe, recurrent **headache** (felt on one or both sides of the head) that is often accompanied by **vomiting** and, in children, by abdominal pain. For this reason, childhood migraine can sometimes be referred to as *abdominal migraine*. Migraine tends to run in families and usually starts in late childhood or in early adolescence. Headaches in children who are younger than this are not usually migraine headaches. It is not yet known what sets off a typical migraine attack, but tension and certain foods, such as cheese, citrus fruit, and chocolate, are all possible culprits. Children can often recover from migraine attacks after vomiting.

Quite often a migraine headache is preceded by an "aura", a series of strange sensations, such as flashing lights, peculiar

POSSIBLE SYMPTOMS

- Severe headache on one or both sides.
- Vomiting.
- Nausea.
- Abdominal pain.
- Paleness.
- Withdrawn, quiet behaviour.
- Aura, involving strange visual and physical sensations, preceding the attack.

smells and numbness on the affected side of the head. Most children can pinpoint these sensations quite clearly.

IS IT SERIOUS?

Migraine is not serious, but it is debilitating.

WHAT SHOULD I DO FIRST?

1 Put your child to bed in a cool, darkened room if he complains of headache and nausea. If the headache persists, it is best to give him a dose of liquid paracetamol.

2 Put a bucket next to your child's bed so that he can vomit without worrying about getting to the toilet in time.

*3 If your child complains of abdominal pain, check him for signs of **appendicitis** (see p. 106).*

SHOULD I CONSULT THE DOCTOR?

Consult your doctor immediately if your child is suffering from severe abdominal pains, to exclude the possibility of appendicitis. Consult your doctor as soon as possible if your child suffers from recurrent migraine headaches.

WHAT MIGHT THE DOCTOR DO?

Your doctor will ask your child to describe the headache. Your doctor may prescribe painkilling drugs for an acute attack. If your child's headaches are frequent, he may be given drugs to take immediately an attack begins or, in severe cases, to be taken regularly to prevent attacks.

WHAT CAN I DO TO HELP?

If the headaches are frequent, keep a diary of your child's diet to try to pinpoint a possible trigger food. Avoid any suspect foods for a couple of weeks to see if there is any reduction in the headaches.

SEE ALSO:
Appendicitis, *page 106*
Headache, *page 116*
Vomiting, *page 100*

MENINGITIS

Meningitis is an inflammation of the membranes (*meninges*) that cover the brain and spinal cord, and most frequently results from an infection, either viral or bacterial. *Viral meningitis* occurs most commonly after **mumps**, but it is not a very serious illness. *Bacterial meningitis*, however, is serious, but can be treated successfully with antibiotics if it is diagnosed early enough. The symptoms of meningitis are **fever**, stiff neck, lethargy, **headache**, drowsiness and intolerance of bright light; in rare cases, there may also be a purple-red rash. Meningitis can be difficult to diagnose in babies and very young children because they are unable to communicate what they are feeling. However, under 18 months old, one noticeable symptom is that the fontanelle will bulge slightly. After that age it closes.

IS IT SERIOUS?

Bacterial meningitis is a very serious disease and, if it is left untreated, it can prove fatal.

POSSIBLE SYMPTOMS

- Fever, as high as 39°C (102.2°F).
- Stiff neck.
- Lethargy and headache.
- Inability to tolerate bright light.
- Bulging fontanelle.
- Drowsiness and confusion.
- Vomiting.
- Purple-red rash anywhere on the body.

COVERINGS OF THE BRAIN

The dura mater, pia mater and the arachnoid membrane are meninges, three membranes that protect the brain.

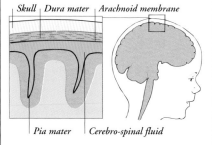

Skull | Dura mater | Arachnoid membrane

Pia mater | Cerebro-spinal fluid

WHAT SHOULD I DO FIRST?

1 If you suspect meningitis, or if he has just had mumps, bend his head forward so that his chin touches his chest to see if there is any stiffness in his neck.

2 If your child is under two years old, check to see if he screws his eyes up in bright light. Feel the fontanelle to see if it bulges outwards.

SHOULD I CONSULT THE DOCTOR?

Consult your doctor immediately if you suspect meningitis.

WHAT MIGHT THE DOCTOR DO?

- If there is any suspicion of meningitis at all, your doctor will refer your child to hospital for a lumbar puncture. This involves removing a sample of spinal fluid, taken under local anaesthetic, for examination.
- If your child is suffering from bacterial meningitis, he will be given high doses of antibiotics intravenously. Viral meningitis clears up on its own, but your child will be given painkilling drugs to relieve the symptoms, and steroids to help recovery.

WHAT CAN I DO TO HELP?

Contact your child's school as meningitis can be contagious.

SEE ALSO:
Fever, *page 25*
Headache, *page 116*
Mumps, *page 29*

CHAPTER

URINARY AND REPRODUCTIVE SYSTEMS

Infections of the urinary and reproductive systems
are common in childhood. They can be distressing
but most clear up quickly. However, you should always
consult your doctor if you are at all worried.
This chapter covers two of the most common
problems, thrush (which is caused by a fungus
and has an anal and vaginal as well as an oral
form) and balanitis, which is the inflammation
of the tip of the penis.

DIAGNOSIS GUIDE

Minor infections of the genitals are quite common in young children and, although they can be distressing, they are not usually serious. To use this section, look for the symptom most similar to the one your child is suffering from, then turn to the relevant entry. See also p. 13 for a list of emergency symptoms.

BOYS' GENITALS

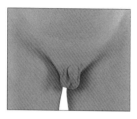

GIRLS' GENITALS

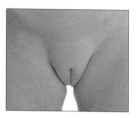

By the time your son is about three or four, the foreskin will be loose and will retract easily. Before that age, you should never try to pull it back for cleaning; just wash the penis carefully. Try to encourage your son to wash the genital area gently from front to back.

Careful hygiene can prevent many genital problems. Teach your little girl to wipe her bottom from front to back so that bacteria from the rectum does not infect the vagina. Scented soap or bubble bath can cause irritation of the genital area, so it is best to use mild, unscented products.

PAIN OR ITCHING in the genital area, *possibly* **Balanitis**, see p. 122

FORESKIN that cannot be drawn back *possibly* **Balanitis**, see p. 122

RED, SWOLLEN TIP of the penis *possibly* **Balanitis**, see p. 122

RED, INFLAMMED BUTTOCKS and genital region *possibly* **Nappy rash**, see p. 49 or **Balanitis**, see p. 122

PIMPLY RED RASH on area normally covered by your baby's nappy *possibly* **Thrush**, see p. 121 or **Nappy rash**, see p. 49

THRUSH

Thrush is a common infection caused by the fungus *Candida albicans*. Under normal circumstances, this fungus is kept under control by other bacteria that also live in the intestines. However, if the balance is disturbed for any reason – for example, when your child is on a course of anti-biotics or his natural resistance is low because of disease – the fungus can grow unchecked, causing infection in any part of the gastro-intestinal tract.

Thrush most often affects the mouth, causing white patches to appear on the tongue, the roof of the mouth and inside the cheeks. It can also affect the anus. In babies, anal thrush is sometimes confused with **nappy rash** because it forms red

patches with little red spots within them. Unlike nappy rash, however, it does not respond to the usual self-help treatments.

POSSIBLE SYMPTOMS

- For oral thrush, creamy yellow or white frothy patches inside the cheeks, on the tongue and the roof of the mouth which become raw or bleed when wiped off.
- A pimply red rash around the anus.

IS IT SERIOUS?

Thrush is rarely serious, but if it does not respond to self-help treatment, get help.

WHAT SHOULD I DO FIRST?

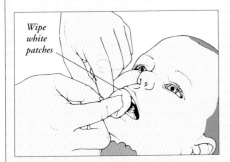

Wipe white patches

1 If your child refuses to eat, check his mouth for any white patches. Try to wipe them off with a handkerchief. If they don't come off or if they leave raw patches underneath, he probably has oral thrush.

2 Avoid giving your child spicy foods and cool all cooked food to lukewarm. Natural yoghurt is the best food to give until you have consulted your doctor.

3 Change your baby's nappies frequently. The fungus may be in his stools and this could give rise to thrush around the anus.

SHOULD I CONSULT THE DOCTOR?

Consult your doctor as soon as possible if you suspect your child has thrush.

WHAT MIGHT THE DOCTOR DO?

- Your doctor will prescribe a liquid anti-fungal medication to be dropped on to the affected area in your child's mouth if he has oral thrush.
- Your doctor will prescribe an anti-fungal cream if there is a rash around the anus.

WHAT CAN I DO TO HELP?

- Feed your child with mild, liquidized foods if he has oral thrush.
- Keep your child's hands clean so that the infection does not spread from the anus to the mouth, or vice versa.
- Leave your baby's bottom exposed to the air as much as possible if he is still in nappies.

SEE ALSO:
Nappy rash, *page 49*

BALANITIS

Balanitis is the inflammation of the tip (*glans*) of the penis. It may be caused by **nappy rash**, by an allergic reaction to the soap powder in which your child's clothes are washed, or by a tight foreskin in boys aged three to five (*phimosis*). Up until then, the foreskin is normally tight.

IS IT SERIOUS?

The condition is not serious, though it is important for your son's comfort that you treat the condition promptly. If it is recurrent, he may need to be circumcised.

POSSIBLE SYMPTOMS

- Red, swollen, moist tip to the penis.
- Discharge of pus from the tip of the penis.
- A foreskin that cannot be drawn back.
- If your child is still in nappies, a general inflammation around the buttocks and in the genital region.

WHAT SHOULD I DO FIRST?

1 As soon as you notice any redness around the tip of the penis, gently try to draw back the foreskin. Don't force it, and leave it if your son is under five. If the foreskin won't retract, leave it alone and consult your doctor as soon as possible.

2 If the foreskin will retract, wash and dry the penis thoroughly and apply an antiseptic ointment.

3 If the condition is part of nappy rash, change your child's nappies frequently, wash and dry the area thoroughly at every nappy change, and apply a barrier cream liberally over the area covered by the nappy, including the penis.

SHOULD I CONSULT THE DOCTOR?

Consult your doctor as soon as possible if your child complains of pain, if you cannot retract the foreskin, or if home treatment fails to relieve the swelling within 48 hours.

WHAT MIGHT THE DOCTOR DO?

- Your doctor may prescribe an antibiotic cream to relieve the inflammation of the penis.

- If the foreskin is tight, your doctor will regularly check on it; if the foreskin has failed to stretch by the time your son is six years old, the condition may need to be corrected surgically by circumcision. Your doctor will refer you to a paediatrician who will assess your child to see if he really needs to be circumcised.

WHAT CAN I DO TO HELP?

- Always change your child's nappies frequently to prevent the recurrence of nappy rash.
- Teach your child good personal hygiene from an early age. Up until the age of five, regular bathing will keep the penis adequately cleaned. After this age, encourage your child to draw back the foreskin and wash the area every day.
- If an allergic reaction has caused balanitis, try changing your washing powder, and make sure that your child's clothing is thoroughly rinsed.

SEE ALSO:

Nappy rash, *page 49*

USEFUL ADDRESSES

If you wish to receive information from any of the organizations listed below, please send a stamped, addressed envelope with your enquiry.

Action for Sick Children
300 Kingston Road
Wimbledon Chase
London SW20 8LX
020 85424848

Pressure group that seeks to raise awareness about the welfare of sick children.

British Dyslexia Association
98 London Road
Reading, Berks. RG1 5AU
0118 9662677

British Red Cross
9 Grosvenor Crescent
London SW1X 7EJ
020 7235 5454

British Stammering Association
15 Old Ford Road
Bethnal Green
London E2 9PJ
Helpline: 020 8983 1003

Contact-a-Family
209–211 City Road
London EC1V 1JN
020 7608 8700

Puts parents of children with special needs in touch with others in their area for support.

MENCAP (The Royal Society for Mentally Handicapped Children and Adults)
Mencap National Centre
123 Golden Lane
London EC1Y 0RT
020 7454 0454

For people with learning disabilities of any kind.

The National Association for Gifted Children (NAGC)
540 Elder House
Milton Keynes MK9 1LR
01908 673677

The National Asthma Campaign
Providence House
Providence Place
London N1 0NT
0845 7010203

The National Deaf Children's Society
15 Dufferin Street
London EC1Y 8UR
020 7250 0123

The National Eczema Society
Hill House
Highgate Hill
London N19 5NA
0870 241 3604

Royal National Institute for the Blind (RNIB)
224 Great Portland Street
London W1N 6AA
020 7388 1266

St. Andrew's Ambulance Association
St Andrew's House
48 Milton Street
Cowcaddans
Glasgow G4 0HR
0141 332 4031

St. John Ambulance
1 Grosvenor Crescent
London SW1X 7EF
0870 2355231

GLOSSARY

Acute
A term applied to short attacks of a disease or pain.

Allergen
A substance which provokes an allergic reaction in certain individuals.

Anaesthetic
A drug used to bring about temporary loss of sensation and hence remove pain. *General anaesthetics* induce unconsciousness and are given in the form of injection or through inhalation, usually for more serious surgical operations. *Local anaesthetics* are usually given as injections and remove sensation from only a limited area. They are used primarily for minor but painful operations.

Analgesic
A pain-relieving drug. The one most frequently given to children is paracetamol, which is available in liquid and tablet form. Paracetamol liquid comes in two strengths: *infants*, from three months to six years, and *junior*, from six to 12 years.

Antibiotic
A drug used to fight bacterial infection. A prescribed course should always be completed, even if the illness is cured.

Antifungal
A drug used to treat fungal infections, such as **thrush** or **athlete's foot**.

Antihistamine
A drug used to counter the effects of histamines, chemicals produced by the body as a result of an allergic, inflammatory reaction. Antihistamine drugs are used to treat illnesses, such as **hives**.

Autoimmune
A defect in the body's defence system against disease, which causes the body to manufacture antibodies that attack and harm its own healthy tissue.

Bacteria
A group of organisms, some of which are harmless and some only harmful when they multiply too quickly. Harmful bacteria can cause illnesses such as **food poisoning** and **tonsillitis**.

Bronchodilator
A drug that widens bronchial passages, and is used in the treatment of **asthma**. It is taken either by nasal inhalation or orally through a spray.

Chronic
A term describing a condition that has lasted, or is expected to last, for some time, while not necessarily being life-threatening.

Excretion
The removal of the body's internal waste matter by natural processes, such as urination and sweating.

Follicle
Most commonly, a tiny cavity on the body's surface.

Hormone
A chemical released by the endocrine glands into the bloodstream. It regulates the activities of certain body organs and tissues.

Immunization
The process by which the body is prepared, by vaccination, to repel any infection or disease.

Incubation period
The interval (measured in days) between the time a disease is caught – when the germs enter the body – and when symptoms appear.

Infection
A type of illness caused by microbes invading the body and multiplying within it. The microbes may clog up blood vessels and ducts, and can also produce harmful waste products.

Laxative
A type of drug used to ease and increase the frequency of bowel movements. They should be given to a child only on doctor's orders.

Membrane
A thin lining or covering tissue of various organs and cavities of the body.

Meninges
The three layers of membrane protecting the brain and spinal cord. **Meningitis** is an inflammation of the meninges.

Microbes
Minute bacteria, viruses or fungi invisible to the naked eye.

Mouth-to-mouth ventilation
An emergency method of reviving someone who is unconscious. It should be given for one minute before calling an ambulance, and started wherever the accident or incident occurred. If you cannot put your mouth over your child's mouth, close off his mouth and breathe into his nose. For babies, it is probably easier to place your mouth over the mouth and nose together. If you are not sure whether you can do this accurately, get emergency instructions by phone while you wait for medical help to arrive.

Mucous membrane
A membrane lining a part of the body, such as the mouth or vagina, which secretes watery or slimy material.

Otoscope
An instrument used to examine the middle and inner ear. It allows the doctor to view through the semi-transparent eardrum, to diagnose disease.

Penicillin
The first antibiotic to be discovered, penicillin is used in the treatment of many infections, including middle ear infection and tonsillitis. It may provoke an allergic reaction. If your child is allergic, make sure this is entered on his medical records and that he wears a medic-alert bracelet so that he isn't given the drug.

Possetting
In babies, the harmless habit of regurgitating milk soon after, or during, a feed.

Pus
A yellow-green substance, made up of decomposed tissue, bacteria and dead white blood cells; it is a sign of the body's fight against infection.

Shock
A reduction of blood flow throughout the body which, if untreated, may lead to collapse, coma and death.

Spasm
An involuntary and uncontrollable contraction of one or more muscles.

Stools
The waste matter left over from food, expelled from the rectum.

Toxin
A poisonous substance produced by bacteria, other microbes and some plants and animals.

Traction
A method of treating broken bones, crushed vertebrae and prolapsed discs. Damaged and compressed parts of the body are held apart by a complex system of pulleys and weights in the correct position until healed.

Ulcer
An open sore affecting either an internal or external body surface.

Vaccine
A solution made up of an altered, weakened or killed strain of a disease. Usually injected, it is designed to stimulate the body's resistance to the disease that has been introduced.

Vasodilator
Any substance, whether a chemical produced by the body, or a drug, which causes blood vessels to widen.

Virus
The smallest type of microbe, which invades the body's cells and multiplies inside them, giving rise to contagious viral infections such as **influenza**.

INDEX

A

abdomen:
  bulges in skin surface, 105
  cramps, 98–99
  pains, 29, 96, 117
acute conditions, 124
adenoids, enlarged, 64
AIDS, 32
allergen, 124
allergic reactions:
  asthma, 90–91
  hayfever, 89
  hives, 53
ambulance, when to call for, 13
anaesthetic, 124
anal fissure, 103
analgesic, 124
anaphylactic shock, 40
angioneurotic oedema, 53
antibiotic, 124
antifungal drugs, 124
antihistamine, 124
appendicitis, 106
appetite, loss of:
  bronchitis, 86
  gastroenteritis, 98
  when to call the doctor, 13
arms, aches and pains, 112
arthritis, 111
asthma, 90–91
athlete's foot, 54
autoimmune system, 124

B

bacteria, 124
balanitis, 122
bites, 37
bleeding wounds, 36
blepharitis, 75
blisters, 41
  on face, 27, 48, 55
  on feet, 41, 54
  small, crops of, 27
blood, on nappy or
  underpants, 103
boil, 47
  gum, 82
bone, broken, 110

diagnosis guide, 108
bowel blockage, 100
bowel motions:
  diagnosis guide, 96
  uncontrollable, 104
breath, unpleasant, 67, 73
breathing difficulties:
  bronchitis, 86
  insect stings, 40
  laboured breathing, 88, 90
bright lights, intolerance of,
  28, 118
broken bone, 110
bronchiolitis, 90
bronchitis, 86
bronchodilator drugs, 91, 124
bruise, 38, 109, 110
burn, 42

C

Candida albicans, 121
catarrh, 64
chapping, 45
chickenpox, 27
chilblains, 46
choking, 92
chronic conditions, 124
circumcision, 122
cold compresses, improvising,
  19
cold-like symptoms, 87, 89,
  93–94
cold sore, 48
cold, 63
colic, 97
common cold, 63
conjunctivitis, 77
constipation, 103, 104, 106
convulsions, 26
cortisone ointment, 49
cot death, 94
coughing, 85
  diagnosis guides, 62, 84
  at night, 64
cradle cap, 50
croup, 88
crying spells, early evening, 97
cuts and grazes, 36
cyanosis, 90

D

dandruff, 57
deafness, 69–70
dehydration, preventing, 21, 101
dental abscesses, 82
depression, 30
developmental delay, 32
diarrhoea, 102
  diagnosis guide, 96
  when to call the doctor, 13
  see also AIDS, 32
diet, high-fibre, 103
digestive complaints, 95–106
  diagnosis guide, 96
dizziness, 115
doctor, when to call, 12–13
drinks, getting a sick child to
  take, 21
drops, administering, 18
drowsiness, 118
dysentry, 98

E, F

ear drops, 18
ears, problems with, 69–72
  diagnosis guide, 62
  earache, 70
  foreign body in, 72
eczema, 51–52
electric shock, 42
emergency, symptoms:
indicating, 13
encephalitis, 27, 29
encopresis, 104
eye drops, 18
eyes, problems with, 75–78
  diagnosis guide, 62
  foreign body in, 78
  see also measles, 28
face, grey or blue colour, 88
  red then blue colour, 92
  swelling, 29, 53
feeding a sick child, 20–21
feet, problems with:
  blisters, 41, 54
  diagnosis guide, 34
  see also toenails and toes
fever, 25–26

diagnosis guide, 25
when to call the doctor, 13, 25–26
first-aid kit, contents of, 19
flea bites, 37
follicle, 124
fontanelle, bulging, 118
food poisoning, 99
foreskin, tight, 122
fractures, bone, 110

G, H

gastroenteritis, 98
genital infections, 119–122
diagnosis guide, 120
German measles, 31
glands, swollen in neck, 30–31, 66–67, 82
glandular fever, 30
glass splinters, 39
glue ear, 69
grazes, 36
growing pain, 112
gum boil, 82
gums, diagnosis guide, 62
haemophilia, 38
hair:
diagnosis guide, 34
washing, 50
hands, problems with:
chapping, 45
chilblains, 46
scabies, 58
hayfever, 89
headache, 116
diagnosis guide, 114
see also chickenpox, 27;
mumps, 29
hearing, loss of, 69–70
heat rash, 44
heatstroke, 43
hernia, 105
Herpes simplex, 48
HIV infection, 32
hives, 53
hoarseness, 68
hormone, 124
hospital:
emergencies requiring, 13
looking after a child in, 22

I, J

immunization, 124
against measles, 28
against tetanus, 37, 39
impetigo, 55
incubation period, 124
infection, 124
infectious diseases, 23–32
diagnosis guide, 24
influenza, 87
ingrowing toenail, 59
insect stings, 40
intussusception, 100
isolating a sick child, 20
itching, 35
diagnosis guide, 34
joints, problems with
diagnosis guide, 108
itchy rash, 58

L, M

laryngitis, 68
laxatives, 103–104, 124
legs, aches and pains, 112
lethargy, 30, 118
leukaemia, 38, 111
lice, 57
limping, 111
lumbar puncture, 118
lymph nodes, enlarged, 32
measles, 28
German, 31
medicines
giving, 16–17
storing, 19
to avoid, 19
meninges, 125
meningitis, 118
migraine, 117
milk regurgitation, 100, 101
mites, 58
mononucleosis, infectious, 30
mouth:
blueness of lips and tongue, 86, 90
ulcers, 81
white or yellow patches inside, 121
white spots inside, 28
mouth-breathing, 67, 89

mouth-to-mouth ventilation, 125
mucous membrane, 125
mumps, 29
muscular pain, 112
muscular weakness, 99

N, O

nails see toenails
nappy rash, 49
nausea, 87, 98, 117
see also vomiting
neck:
blood vessels dilated, 92
stiffness, 118
nervous system complaints, 113–118
diagnosis guide, 114
nettle rash (hives), 53
nits, 57
nose, problems with:
diagnosis guide, 62
foreign body in, 73
nosebleed, 74
nose drops, 18, 64
nursing a sick child, 20–21
occupying a sick child, 21
oral thrush, 49
osteomyelitis, 111
otitis externa, 71
otoscope, 71, 125

P, R

pain and discomfort:
when to call the doctor, 13
penicillin, 125
penis, inflamation of tip, 122
peritonitis, 106
pets, 37, 56
phimosis, 122
pneumonia attack, 32
polyps, nasal, 64
possetting, 100, 101, 125
pus, 125
pyloric stenosis, 101
rashes:
diagnosis guides, 24, 34, 120
heat, 44
nappy, 49
nettle (hives), 53
purple-red (meningitis), 118

respiratory ailments, 83–94
  diagnosis guide, 84
Reye's syndrome, 27, 87
rheumatic fever, 111
ringworm, 56
rotavirus, 98
rubella, 31

S

salivation, 79
salmonella, 99
scabies, 58
scalp problems:
  bald patches, 56
  diagnosis guide, 34
scratching, stopping a child, 35
shock, signs of, 40
sinusitis, 65
skin problems, 34–60
  diagnosis guides, 24, 34, 120
  itching, 35
  see also blisters and rashes
sleeping precautions for babies,
  94
sleeplessness, causes of:
  eczema, 51–52
  growing pain, 112
  teething, 79
  whooping cough, 93
snoring, 67
sore throat, 66
spasms, 125
spleen, enlarged, 30
splinters, 39
splints, improvising, 19
spots see blisters and rashes
sprain, 109
staphylococcus bacterium, 55,
  99

sticky eye, 76
stings, insect, 40
stomach see abdomen
stools, 125
  diagnosis guide, 96
streptococcus bacterium, 55, 66
stye, 75
sudden infant death syndrome
  (SIDS), 94
suffocation, sensation of, 90
sunburn, 43
swallowing, painful, 29
swelling:
  caused by insect stings, 40
  on face, 29, 53
  on neck, 30–31, 66–7, 82
  over bones and joints 38,
    109–110

T

tablets, giving to children, 17
teeth and gums, 79–80, 82
  caring for, 80
  diagnosis guide, 62
teething, 79
temperature, body:
  lowering, 26
  taking, 14–15
  treating raised temperature,
    14–15, 26
  when to call the doctor, 13,
    25–26
testes, swollen and painful, 29
tetanus, 37, 39
thermometers, 14–15
throat problems, 66–68
  diagnosis guide, 62
  grasping by child, 92
  sore throat, 66

thrush, 121
  oral, 49
toenails
  cutting, 59
  ingrowing, 59
  thick yellow, 54
toes, problems with
  itchy rash, 58
  white blistered skin, 54
tonsillitis, 67
tooth decay, preventing, 80
toothache, 80
traction, 125
travel sickness, 100

U, V, W

ulcer, 125
  mouth, 81
urticaria (hives), 53
vaccine, 125
vasodilator, 46, 125
verruca, 60
voice, loss of, 68
vomiting, 100–101
  diagnosis guide, 100
  helping a child, 20
  when to call the doctor, 13
  see also bronchitis, 86;
    catarrh, 64; hernia, 105;
    influenza, 87; whooping
    cough, 93
weals, 53
weeping blister, 48
weight loss in babies:
  inexplicable, 94
wheezing, 88, 90
whooping cough, 93
withdrawn behaviour, 117
wounds, 36–37

ACKNOWLEDGMENTS

Dorling Kindersley would like to
thank the following individuals and
organizations for their contribution
to this book.

EDITORIAL ASSISTANCE
Nicky Adamson, Caroline Greene,
Maureen Rissik

PICTURES
Science Photo Library (pp. 29, 53)

INDEX
Robert Hood

TEXT FILM
Brightside Partnership,
London